Instant Medical Adviser

Instant answers to more than
300 medical diseases or problems

plus

Emergency First Aid Guide

Food Guide including reducing diets, crash and formula
diets, typical diets, and diets for children

Illustrated Exercise Charts

Complete Alphabetical Index

1994 Edition

© Copyright 1994 by

CAREER PUBLISHING, INC.

Library of Congress Catalog Card No. 77-137377
Printed in the United States of America
All rights reserved

ISBN   0-911744-08-8

MA94-1

Purpose of This Book

This Instant Medical Adviser provides in compact form authoritative information about more than 300 medical problems, diseases, and emergencies. The book is especially designed to answer the medical questions most frequently asked and to provide the information most often needed.

Main subjects are alphabetically arranged so that they may be quickly found without referring to the index. However, sub-topics which may be discussed under a main heading can readily be found by use of the index. For example, *Hay Fever* is a form of *Allergy* and is discussed under that main subject. By looking under *Hay Fever* in the index, you would immediately find the proper page reference.

In addition to the informative articles, the *Instant Medical Adviser* contains an illustrated program of warm-up exercises and an illustrated series of reducing and conditioning exercises. Also included in this handy volume are other programs and schedules for maintaining good health as well as useful medical checklists, charts and diagrams.

For fast use in emergencies, a comprehensive *First Aid Guide* is included. This easy-to-use guide indicates proper care for minor emergencies plus what to do in case of more serious emergencies while awaiting the physician. The Guide can save important moments and provide information on proper care at a time when it is most needed.

ABDOMEN, DISTENDED   Enlargement of structures within the abdomen will lead to distention, a bulging contour. By far the most common cause of this is pregnancy. By the end of the third month, the pregnant uterus has grown out of the pelvic cavity and may be felt just above the pelvic bones in the bladder region. By the sixth month, the pregnant uterus has reached the level of the umbilicus; by the ninth month, it is close to the lowermost portion of the breastbone. The only comparable enlargement is that found with certain very large cysts of the ovary. In the course of such abdominal enlargement there may be a stretching and cracking of the connective tissue of the skin resulting in linear markings over the lower abdomen known as striae; these generally appear pink during pregnancy, but afterwards turn white. During a succeeding pregnancy new pink markings dispersed among the older ones may be seen. Neither abdominal supports nor other measures will prevent such markings. The number vary from individual to individual. There are some who never show striae, or in whom they are inconspicuous.

ABDOMINAL PAINS   Most of the important abdominal organs have muscles in their walls. Food and wastes are moved along by contractions of these muscles, but ordinarily one is not aware of such muscular activity. However, when inflammation or obstruction is present, severe and painful contractions may occur. These pains generally come and go rhythmically, may mount in intensity and then decrease somewhat, and are often referred to as painful spasms, colic, or griping pains.

Severe colicky pains may be experienced with the movement of gallstones or urinary stones, or when intestinal obstruction is present. The pain of appendicitis often starts as a colicky pain perhaps due to obstruction in the canal within the appendix. Colicky pains felt in the lower abdomen preceding a bowel movement, as in dysentery and diarrhea, generally point to involvement of the large intestine. In certain disorders the pain may also be felt in the back and occasionally may radiate to other parts of the body. Thus the pain of gallbladder disease may be felt not only in the back but also in the right shoulder, and occasionally a kidney stone may produce pain which shoots down to the groin and upper thigh.

Sometimes the pain of inflammation within the abdomen is a steady one. This is true in appendicitis once the initial crampy pains have subsided. The pain then experienced will be a localized pain in the region of the appendix itself. A somewhat similar course of events may occur in inflammation of the gallbladder, the pancreas, the colon, and other organs. Often such pain is accompanied by nausea and sometimes by vomiting. In addition, a few points to remember about abdominal pain are:

1. Never assume that abdominal pain is due to constipation nor take a laxative when you are experiencing pain, unless so directed by a doctor.

2. Most forms of abdominal pain can be helped to some degree by heat, as by a heating pad.

3. Abdominal pain is only a symptom: an explanation for it should be forthcoming. Check it out with the doctor. Thus in pregnancy acute appendicitis may produce atypical abdominal pains felt in a location higher or different from the usual one. Sometimes a blood count or other special tests may be necessary to determine the cause of any particular pain. (See also APPENDICITIS.)

ABORTION   An abortion is properly defined as any interruption in a pregnancy prior to the time that the fetus (unborn child) can live independently—that is, about the sixth month.

▶ **Spontaneous abortion** (often referred to as a miscarriage) may result from any number of conditions, some of which are identifiable, others not. Falls or blows to the abdomen, a severe febrile illness such as influenza or typhoid fever, or operative procedures are sometimes the cause. Very often no cause is found, although careful study sometimes indicates that the embryo was abnormal. Spontaneous abortion is by no means rare; perhaps one in every four or five pregnancies will result in such an abortion. One uncertainty in estimating their number is the fact that abortion early in pregnancy may be difficult to recognize. It is quite likely that some of the delayed periods reported by women represent an early and unrecognized abortion. A small but distressing percentage of women may abort with virtually every pregnancy. They are sometimes referred to as "chronic aborters." In most instances the reasons for this are not understood. Occasionally the pregnancy may be carried to term by bedrest, hormone administration, removal of fibroids, and other measures.

▶ **Therapeutic abortion** is one performed for a sound medical reason, as for instance psychiatric disease, German measles (in the first three months of pregnancy), active tuberculosis, certain cardiac conditions, and other disturbances. A therapeutic abortion is generally performed in a hospital setting, requires the signature of at least two doctors, and is a safe procedure ordinarily.

▶ **Criminal abortion** is an illegal operation for terminating pregnancy. It is often performed surreptitiously, and not always in the cleanliest or most skillful fashion. Some risk may therefore be attached to it, despite which it has been estimated that as many as a million such operations are performed per year.

▶ **Induced abortion** is a general term for an abortion produced by some procedure or drug. In fact, however, most drugs used to stimulate the uterus to evacuate its contents are singularly unsuccessful.

ABSCESS   An abscess is any localized collection of pus in the body. An abscess forms as a result of invasion by bacteria or other organisms, with consequent breakdown of tissue. Abscesses are often described in terms of their locations. Thus an *appendiceal abscess* is one occurring within the abdominal cavity in close relation to the appendix, and generally subsequent to a ruptured appendix, i.e., appendicitis.

A *lung abscess* frequently follows an inflammation in the lung caused by certain organisms such as the staphylococcus, or as a result of violent mixed infections that may occur if vomited material is aspirated into the lungs.

Boils and carbuncles are essentially abscesses within the skin. Since they normally come to a "head," thereby instituting drainage (which is desirable in healing), they pose less of a threat than similar kinds of inflammations in the organs.

Breast abscess, a fairly common form of abscess, occurs in the tissue of the breast; this is seen most often in post-partum women and in nursing mothers. Most of these abscesses are due to an invasion of the breast tissue by skin organisms which either enter via some minute crack in the nipple or work their way down through the breast duct system. A breast abscess manifests itself as a warm tender swelling, sometimes accompanied by chills or fever. It may respond to local compresses and antibiotics by mouth. If it does not, the swelling will continue and may become fluctuant (soft), at which point an incision to produce drainage may be necessary. Once drainage is established, the abscess empties itself and healing generally occurs without incident.

A *pelvic abscess* is one which forms in the pelvic cavity and is often secondary to inflammations of a pelvic organ. Inflammations of the tube and ovary may lead to this, but so also may inflammations of the large intestine. Suppuration of the appendix may also drain off into the pelvic cavity and produce an abscess there.

ACQUIRED IMMUNE DEFICIENCY SYNDROME (AIDS) AIDS results from infection by HTLV-III virus that is associated with debilitating, and often fatal diseases. A great deal of fear and anxiety results from misinformation or lack of information. Many thousands of cases of AIDS have been reported and the number increases each year. Those at high risk are homosexual/bisexual men, parenteral (intravenous) drug users, and hemophiliacs.

Surveillance of known cases suggest a pattern of transmission resembling that of hepatitis B virus by blood and body fluids. Researchers agree on the routes of transmission: sexual, intravenous transfusion of blood and blood products, and mother to fetus. What is unknown is which cofactors make an infected host more likely to develop the complications of AIDS. It is believed that AIDS occurs only in persons whose immune systems are already vulnerable.

Sexual transmission is the most common cause of acquiring AIDS, and the greatest risk of transmission is among homosexual men. Heterosexual transmission has been apparent since the beginning of the epidemic, though the incidence is relatively low. Male-to-female transmission may be the most common (rather than female-to-male) since semen can carry infected lymphocytes. Most of the evidence is

8

based on patients who have had sustained or recurrent relationships with a person with AIDS or a person in a high incidence group, or who has had multiple sexual contacts. Multiple sexual contacts place both heterosexual men and women at risk.

To avoid acquiring AIDS, emphasis is placed on the importance of knowing one's partner and practicing healthy sex which means no exchange of body fluids (including semen, urine, saliva, feces, or blood), or contact of body fluids with mucous membranes. Attention to risk reducing behavior is most important even among persons who already are infected.

ALCOHOL SPONGE RUB (BATH) An alcohol sponge rub is a rapid way of lowering the body temperature during high fevers. It will also remove accumulated skin oils and perspiration. By killing surface bacteria it also has a disinfectant action.

A properly conducted alcohol sponge rub will lower body temperature by several degrees within half an hour, but care to avoid chilling should be exercised. If the patient complains of chilliness, it is probably best to stop the sponging. Other precautions are to avoid getting alcohol fumes into the eyes and to bypass the face, and the anal and genital areas.

Sponging can be done with straight rubbing alcohol, or with a mixture of half alcohol and half tepid water. (The latter is less drying and less chilling.)

In addition to a basin with alcohol, one will need two washcloths and one or two large towels. A light blanket (or bath towel) can be used for covering the patient during the procedure. One should be sure to protect any furniture against splashing with alcohol since it may spoil the finish. Newspapers or plastic covers will be helpful.

An alcohol sponge rub is performed as follows:

1. Bring the patient toward the side of the bed.
2. Remove gown or pajamas.
3. Wring out one washcloth in the alcohol or alcohol-water mixture and place on the abdomen; renew frequently throughout the procedure.
4. Dip the other washcloth in alcohol and in rotation sponge

9

the arms, the trunk and the legs. Place a bath towel under each part being sponged to protect the bedding.

5. Turn the patient over and sponge the back; this may be followed up with rubbing in a body lotion.

6. Spend about five minutes each on the arms, chest, and the legs.

7. Check temperature in a half hour.

ALLERGY   Allergy is a condition of hypersensitivity or altered tissue reactivity. Antigens (sensitizing agents) are found in various foods, bacteria, drugs, medications, pollens (inhalants). These sensitizing agents produce antibodies in the blood of allergic people. As a consequence of antigen-antibody reaction, certain symptoms occur. These can resemble common colds with running nose, sneezing, watering of the eyes; colic with abdominal pains, distention, gas; croup with wheezing, cough, rashes, bronchitis, stomach aches, vomiting, itchy sensations, etc.

More than half of all allergic symptoms are found in the first few years of childhood. They can appear in any organ of the body, but are most common in those systems where there is exposure to foreign substances, such as the respiratory tract, the skin, and the gastrointestinal tract. With young infants who are on a limited diet, it may be relatively easy to determine what foods cause allergy in the first few months of life. If an infant breaks out with a skin rash soon after being introduced to orange juice, egg, or a cereal, it is possible to assume that one of them is the allergic substance. One may then withdraw the food from the diet, use ointments to clear the rash, and observe the patient. If the rash does not recur after the offending food has been eliminated, it is good evidence that the food was causing the allergic response.

In some children there is a history of "keeping a cold all winter long," of wheezing the minute they get outside into the cold air, and inability to take a bath without catching cold the following morning (presumably due to exposure with a change in temperature). These children are sometimes also unable to go swimming in the summer because the chilling water and change of temperature predisposes them to catching cold. These may be signs of upper-respiratory infection allergy and may be associated with wheezing and a clinical picture resembling asthma. While this may not be true asthma, it is considered

10

asthmatic bronchitis because it occurs whenever the child has some slight chilling or upper-respiratory infection. These children are frequently allergic to bacteria. The onset of a cold triggers a wheezing episode. They can usually be treated and desensitized with a respiratory vaccine. This causes a reduction in the frequency, severity, and duration of these symptoms. (See also Asthma.)

► **Drug Allergy** Many persons are sensitive to the chemicals in drugs. This reaction is not caused by an overdose but by a particular sensitivity. Children, in particular, may have an unexpected reaction to a medication—an effect quite opposite to what was intended. For instance, if the drug is a sedative, the child may become excited and agitated. Children often do not respond to many preparations which are designed to cure their illness.

Symptoms. The symptoms produced by drug allergy reaction are usually the same as those produced by pollen, house dust, food, inhalants, or other substances. There may be swelling of the mucous membranes of the nose and throat, hives, rashes, headache, mental dullness, wheezing, etc.

Treatment. Treatment involves eliminating these particular medications. Adrenalin and cortisone may also be used.

► **Gastrointestinal Allergy** The symptoms of this form of allergic reaction are: headaches, vomiting, diarrhea, and recurring abdominal pain. Small infants may have repeated bouts of vomiting if they are allergic to cow's milk protein. Their stools may become loose and watery. They may tense up and cry with pain, indicating colic. They may also break out with various skin rashes, such as hives, or have eczema or generalized itching without any evidence of rash.

For infants and children the most frequent allergenic foods are: cow's milk, orange juice, tomatoes and tomato juice, chocolate, eggs, fish, nuts, and the various citrus fruits. Children who are allergic to one of these may frequently be sensitive to all of them.

Treatment. Treatment depends upon finding the food or drink which causes the reaction. Attacks may be relieved by eliminating these foods and by giving injections of adrenalin. Antihistamines may also be of help.

► **Serum Sickness** Serum sickness is a response to certain injections which contain horse serum. The patient may be allergic to certain immunization procedures and should be tested before receiving them. Injection material made from horse serum, or incubated on egg yolk, may cause sensitivity. The symptoms are headache, nausea, vomiting and fever, and hives, with swelling of the glands. Joints may become swollen and painful. The treatment is adrenalin, antihistamines, and cortisone.

► **Hay Fever** This disorder is due to a state of allergy or hypersensitivity primarily involving the nose and eyes, producing cold-like symptoms. The usual complaints are of nasal congestion, watery secretion, sneezing, itching of the eyes, and tearing. Predisposition is inherited: a hay fever sufferer will generally be found to have one or more close relatives (his parents, brothers and sisters, or aunts and uncles) who share the same discomfort. Hypersensitivity is most often to the pollens of certain grasses, trees, and weeds—although not infrequently multiple sensitivities exist, such as allergic reactions to dusts, bacterial infections, and/or various food items.

A normal individual can inhale air containing large amounts of ragweed pollen with no reaction whatsoever. In contrast, the hay fever victim will show immediate reactions of the sort mentioned earlier. Because of the sensitivity, there is local production in the tissues of a chemical called histamine. Histamine results in prompt swelling and inflammation. Its production in the tissues will go on quite continuously throughout the time of exposure, which in the case of the ragweed season generally runs from about mid-August until the first frost. The existence of the excessive sensitivity can also be shown by appropriate skin tests. Injection of a tiny amount of even very diluted extracts of the offending agents will produce a marked skin reaction in the sensitized individual.

Various methods are available for the treatment of hay fever:

1. In desensitization, progressively increasing amounts of the extract of the offending substances are injected under the skin.

2. A group of drugs known as the antihistamines seem to neutralize or antagonize the local effects of histamine.

3. Steroid (cortisone-type) drugs have as one of their general properties the ability to abolish reactions of hypersensitivity.

4. Drugs related to atropine and ephedrine may also have a marked drying effect on the swollen, congested nasal linings.

12

5. A change of location to a low pollen count area may give the hay fever victim relief.

▶ **Testing for Allergy** An allergic child or adult should have a complete physical examination, history, and laboratory tests, such as blood count, urinalysis, and nasal smear. Following this there are three types of skin tests which can be performed to determine the allergies.

The most frequently used is the *scratch test* in which a small amount of specific substance is introduced onto the skin and a small scratch made, usually on the forearm. If a small wheal (which looks like a small mosquito bite) develops, this is a suspicious, positive reaction to the allergen in question. Some patients may show a positive skin-test reaction to substances which they have never eaten or been exposed to. Such a reaction does not necessarily indicate that they are allergic to these substances.

An *intradermal test* is one in which the antigen is injected into the dermal (deeper) layer of the skin with a tiny needle. This test is more sensitive and may give a strongly positive reaction if the person is allergic to the material. A *patch test,* in which the allergic material is placed on the skin as a sort of patch and left for twenty-four to forty-eight hours, is another method of testing for sensitivity.

Passive transfer is a special method which is used when the skin cannot be involved in testing, as in severe eczema, or with children who are too difficult to test. It is also used to spare the individual the test procedures. The serum obtained from the allergic person is injected into the skin of a number of areas of a normal person. A few days later the allergic extracts are introduced into the same areas on the skin and the tests are read.

Allergy can also be tested by placing a drop of antigen into the eye of a sensitive person. The reaction is noted by comparing it with the response to a normal control.

ALZHEIMER'S DISEASE (AD) *What is Alzheimer's Disease?* Alzheimer's Disease is a progressive disorder of the brain causing loss of memory or serious mental deterioration. Little is known about the cause of this disorder, but research shows that nerve endings in the cortex of the brain degenerate and disrupt the passage of electrochemical signals between the cells.

What are the symptoms? There are many patterns in the type, severity, and sequence of mental changes in AD. Usually, the symptoms are progressive but vary greatly in the rate of change from person to person. In a few cases, there may be rapid mental deterioration, but often, there are long periods in which little change is noted. However, the progressive deterioration which occurs is a source of deep concern and frustration for both the victim and the family.

As the disease progresses, the changes in the nerve cells produce simple forgetfulness and increasingly more noticable memory loss. Changes in thought, language, personality, and behavior can eventually render the person incapable of taking care of himself or communicating his needs to others.

What is the Treatment? Medical care can *relieve many of the symptoms* of AD but prevention or cure of the disease is not known. Counseling can help the victim and his family in coping with the illness. A neurologist, psychiatrist, or family physician should closely monitor treatment and have the time and interest to answer the variety of questions that arise. Medication can be prescribed to improve sleeping patterns. Proper nutrition, exercise and physical therapy can aid difficulties that arise in physical functioning. Social contacts should be encouraged. A list of daily tasks, written reminders, and safety measures can assist the individual in day-to-day living. It is best to maintain an ordered environment so that the afflicted person does not have to continuously learn new things.

ANEMIA   The function of the red blood cells is to carry oxygen and nutrition to the tissues and carbon dioxide from the tissues. The main element of red blood cells is hemoglobin, which is made from stores of iron and protein in the body. These are derived from food and from the destruction of hemoglobin in the body for the iron is reused.

Anemia is a lowering of the red blood cells, or hemoglobin, below the normal value for the age of the person. It may or may not produce symptoms such as fatigue, weakness, or headaches. The diagnosis of anemia is made by drawing a drop of blood from the finger, diluting it in a standard solution, and examining and counting the cells directly under a microscope. The cells are also stained with dye and the colors and shapes examined on a slide. A defect of the red blood cells, or hemoglobin, reflects a disturbance of the production of iron, or a loss or destruction of these elements.

▶ **Anemias of Pregnancy** Anemia is a good deal more common in women than in men, due to the loss of iron women experience with each menstrual period. Anemia is therefore more likely to develop with heavy and frequent periods.

Pregnancy may be another contributory factor, for the developing baby will draw on maternal iron stores. It is quite common, therefore, to prescribe iron supplements during pregnancy. Prenatal vitamin supplements often have calcium and iron added to them in recognition of the extra need for these two elements. Although, as a rule, blood loss at the time of delivery creates no problem, it may be sufficient to result in mild anemia. In such an event the doctor will probably prescribe iron supplements to be taken for some time after the delivery. As can be seen, the crucial factor in most of the anemias that affect women is the availability of iron.

There are some rare anemias in pregnancy known as megaloblastic anemias. These are not due to iron deficiency but rather to an inadequate supply of folic acid, a member of the B group of vitamins; the condition is remedied by giving folic acid by injection. Occasionally also, considerable amounts of bleeding from hemorrhoids or from disorders not necessarily associated with pregnancy (such as a bleeding peptic ulcer) may contribute to anemia. Occurrences of this sort should be reported to the doctor who will in any case routinely check for anemia in pregnancy.

▶ **Hemolytic Anemias** These anemias refer to destruction *within the bloodstream* of the red blood cells. They may be due to congenital or hereditary disorders which result in defects in the production of red blood cells and/or hemoglobin. As the red blood cells are destroyed, part of the hemoglobin is released from these cells and the bile pigment (bilirubin) formed leads to an increase in the bilirubin level in the blood. This eventually gives a yellowish color to the skin called

15

jaundice. In severe, chronic, hemolytic anemias, there may also be an accumulation of iron-containing pigment in the body tissues, leading to an enlargement of the liver and a characteristic gray-green discoloration of the skin.

In some of these anemias the spleen, which is the main organ for the destruction of the blood, is often enlarged, and one may be able to feel its outlines in the abdomen.

▶ **Iron Deficiency Anemia** This is due to deficient or poor nutrition, chronic illness, or excess loss of iron. The red cells are usually small (microcytic) and are filled with very small amounts of hemoglobin, indicating that they are hypochromic (without much color).

The symptoms of this anemia are varied, and may include poor appetite, decrease in normal activity, irritability, behavior disorders, pale skin. The poor appetite leads to a further poor intake of iron and exaggerates the degree of anemia. The condition is slowly progressive and may lead to serious disorders of the heart and respiration. It should, therefore, be corrected as soon as possible. The patient must be supplied with food rich in iron, or with medications, sometimes called "tonics," containing iron salts. Periodic blood counts should be taken to indicate the progress of the anemia or its correction. (See also BLOOD.)

APPENDICITIS The appendix is a small, dead-end pouch, situated just below the point where the small intestine empties into the large; it is, therefore, located in the right lower fourth of the abdomen. The appendix performs no useful digestive function, its chief importance arising from the fact that it occasionally becomes inflamed—appendicitis—and can pose a threat of serious and spreading infection within the abdomen.

Although appendicitis is generally regarded as a disease of children and young adults, it can occur in all age groups, including the elderly. Its symptoms may be deceptively mild, particularly at the beginning, and can easily be dismissed as "an upset stomach." Typically, it starts with cramping abdominal pains experienced in the upper abdomen, generally above the level of the "belly button" (navel). There is usually an associated loss of appetite which may progress to nausea and occasionally to vomiting. Over the course of the next six

16

to twelve hours there is increasing localization of pain in the abdominal region of the appendix.

The appendix is inches below and to the right of the navel. The pain here will be steady, and will increase if the patient coughs or is asked to "blow out" the abdomen. When the doctor makes his examination, he will look for such signs as:

1. *Tenderness* to pressure in the area.

2. *Guarding*—involuntary tightening up of the abdominal muscle overlying the inflamed appendix.

3. *Rebound*—the sudden sharp increase in pain produced when manual pressure in this region is suddenly released.

There may not always be certainty in diagnosing acute appendicitis; among some of the conditions that imitate it are ovulation with the release of an egg and certain inflammations, generally viral, of the abdominal lymph glands. It may therefore be considered wise to hospitalize a suspected case of appendicitis for repeated blood cell counts and observations before the diagnosis can be established.

Treatment. There are no first-aid measures of any value in appendicitis. An icebag placed over the region may produce some relief of pain. Nothing should be given by mouth. Above all *be sure to avoid the use of laxatives.* It is a grievous error to mistake acute appendicitis as "gas pains" or "spastic constipation" and take a laxative, for this may produce rupture of the inflamed appendix and a spreading peritonitis. Clearly, both diagnosis and treatment require the skill of a doctor, who must check the patient. Remember that there are unusual cases of appendicitis in which the person feels "a little sick," has a little soreness over the region of the appendix, and yet proves to have a severely inflamed appendix when surgery is performed. The degree of inflammation cannot be judged by fever; this seldom exceeds 100°F. by mouth throughout the early stages.

▶ **Mesenteric Adenitis** A non-surgical condition which resembles appendicitis is called mesenteric adenitis. The mesentery is a lining covering the intestines. It contains blood vessels and lymph glands. When acute infection exists, such as in cases of tonsillitis, bronchitis, pneumonias, etc., these abdominal glands may become swollen, tender, and painful, causing nausea, vomiting and abdominal pain. It resembles acute appendicitis very closely. However, antibiotic treatment of the general infection will usually make these glands subside and the symptoms will disappear. In true acute appendicitis the symptoms usually do not disappear. However, in many cases, surgical intervention may be necessary because of the danger of missing an acute appendix. (See also ABDOMINAL PAINS.)

ARTERIES, HARDENING OF (ATHEROSCLEROSIS)

This is by far the most common and most important abnormal condition found in the human body. The basic process consists of deposits of fatty materials which are readily visible as yellow streaks and mounds in the inner lining of the arteries. The deposits tend to be irregular in extent and location; they can be present to an excessive degree in one location, as for example, in the coronary arteries of the heart, with only slight-to-moderate involvement elsewhere.

When it is widespread and advanced, the condition is sometimes spoken of as "generalized arteriosclerosis;" disorders produced by this condition are traceable to impairment of the circulation. Decreased circulation results from the fatty deposits, which encroach on the caliber of the blood vessel. In addition, there is a local slowing of the bloodstream, which can result in the formation of thromboses or clots. When this occurs in an artery of the heart, a coronary thrombosis (heart attack) is the result; if the vessel involved happens to be one in the brain, a stroke (with paralysis) may result. If the clot is in an important vessel going to the lower extremities, death (gangrene) of the tissue there will follow.

It was formerly thought that atherosclerosis was a normal aging phenomenon in arteries. It is now regarded as a disease process which tends to increase with aging but which is variable and partially, if not largely, preventable. Many factors can contribute to the degree of atherosclerosis, although there is uncertainty about their relative importance. Some of these are:

1. The level of such *blood fats* as the neutral fats called triglycerides and the waxlike fat called cholesterol; when these are elevated, the degree of atherosclerosis is increased. (See CHOLESTEROL.)

2. *High blood pressure,* which tends to increase atherosclerosis.

18

3. *Sex hormones.* All else being equal, female sex hormone protects against, and male sex hormone tends to favor, atherosclerosis. Hence, till the menopause, the female has a distinct advantage over the male in this respect.

4. *High saturated-fat diets.* It appears that diets in which the saturated fats are reduced and the polyunsaturated fats increased may favorably affect atherosclerosis.

5. *Cigarette smoking.* This appears to increase the likelihood of coronary thrombosis—presumably by some effect on atherosclerosis there.

6. *Metabolic disorders* such as diabetes and hypothyroidism. These significantly increase the rate of atherosclerosis.

The possibility that atherosclerosis may be controllable by diet has excited widespread attention and has resulted in a changing pattern in the fat consumption of Americans. Probably overweight also tends to increase atherosclerosis. (See also CORONARY THROMBOSIS.)

ARTHRITIS   Most bones of the body interact with others at a site called the joint. Most joints are so constructed as to permit some freedom of motion; this freedom may be very extensive (as in the shoulder or the elbow) or quite restricted (as in the joints found in the spinal column). In many, though not all, joints the bony surface concerned is covered by a layer of cartilage (gristle) and the joint may have a special delicate lining (the synovium).

Diseases of the joints are termed "arthritis." Despite their relatively simple structure, the joints are involved in a great many local and general disorders. Some are related to the allergic disorders, as is seen in the acute arthritis of rheumatic fever or of a penicillin reaction. Damage to a joint, as through a fall or blow, may produce fractures in the bones, as well as a filling-up of the joint with an increased amount of secretion; this is spoken of as traumatic arthritis. In gout, deposits of a chemical (uric acid) may occur in and about the joints, leading to the condition known as gouty arthritis.

It is also important to know that not all of the pains and discomforts around joints are due to arthritis; many are due to disorders of the muscular tendons and are known as *tendonitis.* (Tendonitis in the shoulder joint is frequently referred to as "Charley-horse.") The two major forms of arthritis

19

which must be reckoned with are osteoarthritis and rheumatoid arthritis.

▶ **Osteoarthritis** Osteoarthritis, a disorder that almost everyone will experience as he gets older, is marked by a proliferation of the bone at the joint site. This is of very variable degree. Minor forms of osteoarthritis produce no symptoms or discomfort. The thickening of the finger joints seen in many individuals past age fifty is an example of this form of arthritis. In a small percentage, thickening leads to deformity and moderate amounts of pain, the latter most likely to be experienced on arising in the morning. Other joints that may be involved in osteoarthritis in the elderly are the hip and the knee —the more so if overweight is present. Symptoms include mild achiness and stiffness which are made worse by resting or by exposure to cold. Other common sites at which osteoarthritis occurs are the joints of the spine, the shoulders, and the elbows. When necessary, the condition is treated by such simple drugs as aspirin and its derivatives, and by local heat.

▶ **Rheumatoid arthritis** is a far more serious and crippling condition. This probably represents a chronic allergic type of disorder involving the joints with production of increased fluid, heat, and pain. Sometimes all the major joints are attacked to produce generalized or disseminated rheumatoid arthritis. In other instances (especially in the early stages) the spine alone, or only the hands and the feet, are attacked. Neither the basic nature of nor basic therapy for rheumatoid arthritis is yet known. Immediate control of even severe rheumatoid arthritis can be secured by the use of steroid drugs (cortisone-type drugs). Other treatments that have been used include injections of gold and such drugs as aspirin and butazolidine, perhaps supplemented by such pain-killing agents as the codeine group of drugs. Many doctors rely heavily on physical therapy. Rheumatoid arthritis must be regarded as a troublesome affliction which can be helped—but not cured. The patient must learn to live with the disease and do what he can despite it.

ARTIFICIAL RESPIRATION

(1) CLEAN MOUTH AND EXTEND HEAD

(2) PULL JAW FORWARD AND PINCH NOSTRILS

(3) BLOW AIR INTO MOUTH. CHEST SHOULD RISE

21

ARTIFICIAL RESPIRATION   Artificial respiration should be used on anyone whose breathing is greatly slowed or stopped; this includes victims of poisoning, drowning, and accidents. All previous methods of artificial respiration have now been replaced by the mouth-to-mouth method, which is performed as follows:

1. Clear the victim's mouth of any dirt, sand, clothing, or other foreign matter.

2. Place the victim flat on his back with head extended. Kneel alongside, at the victim's shoulder level. With the fingers of one hand hook the under-surface of the victim's jaw and pull on it so that it juts forward.

3. Press your mouth against the victim's mouth so as to form a relatively airtight connection. With a small child, the rescuer's mouth should cover both the victim's mouth and nose. With an adult, the rescuer should pinch the victim's nostrils together with his free hand.

4. Blow air into the victim's mouth with quick, deep puffs, as in blowing out a candle. (The puffs are bigger for an adult than for a child and should produce movement of the victim's chest like that in deep breathing.) Repeat twelve to fifteen times per minute for an adult, up to twenty times per minute for a child.

5. Allow the lungs of the victim to deflate between breaths. (Gentle pressure with one hand on the victim's abdomen will help deflation.)

6. Artificial respiration should be maintained *without halt* until a physician arrives at the scene or while transporting the patient to a hospital. (See also drawing on page 21.)

ASTHMA   The bronchial tubes have muscles in their walls which can contract, thus narrowing the size of the tube. Excessive degrees of contraction of the bronchial muscle is referred to as bronchospasm; much of the difficulty that occurs in asthma is traceable to bronchospasm. If, in addition, there is accumulated secretion within the bronchial tube, the difficulty in getting air in and out may become marked. An obvious wheezing is often noted and the emptying of air out of the lungs (normally an easy process not requiring any effort) may be difficult and prolonged. All of this to a lesser or greater degree is observed in asthma. Even in moderate degrees of asthma the effort of breathing may be painful to behold. The victim has to labor to get air in and out, and like anyone else who is working hard may be drenched in perspiration.

Most cases of asthma are due to allergy, that is, a hypersensitivity to some offending substance. In the most common type, that due to pollens, the disease is often combined with hay fever. (This form of asthma is also known as seasonal asthma.) A good guess as to the cause may be based on observation of the time that the disease is active, and a knowledge of the local pollens. Thus, asthma that occurs in the spring is generally due to the pollens of the grasses and trees, while the common asthma that starts in the late summer or early fall is generally traceable to ragweed. Sometimes molds and dust may be at fault; less often, an allergic response to something that the person has eaten may produce asthma.

In another form of the disease the asthmatic response seems to be brought about by bronchitis, the sensitivity apparently being due to bacteria or their products associated with the bronchitis. This is known as *asthmatoid bronchitis*. It is more likely to come on in the middle years (as compared to ordinary asthma which appears earlier in life), is made worse by respiratory infections, and may be present all year 'round.

Treatment. There are various approaches a doctor may use in the treatment of asthma: (1) desensitization to the offending agent, (2) bronchodilator drugs, or (3) steroid drugs. (See also ALLERGY; BRONCHITIS.)

BABY-SITTERS   There are about a million persons who do baby-sitting in the United States. Most baby-sitters are teen-agers and fortunately they usually like youngsters, but the parent must remember that a baby-sitter is not the parent and therefore there are definite limits that must be set for the baby-sitter. Baby-sitters should not be asked to perform the functions of a nurse or doctor.

A new baby-sitter should be given an orientation talk which will include information about what the child likes, how the home is run, situations the baby-sitter is to be particularly alerted to, especially those that are likely to result in accidents. But, of course, the most important lesson you must get across to the baby-sitter is that his or her main job is to watch the child, so that you will find your child safe when you return home.

When you have special instructions, *put them in writing.* Such writing should include your policy of not permitting the baby-sitter to have visitors or to monopolize the telephone. Write out very clearly specific or extra chores that you may want the baby-sitter to perform. Of course other information should be written down, and this includes the following:

Important Telephone Numbers:

Where parents can be reached_____

Where doctor can be reached_____

Close friend or neighbor_____

Police Department: Dial "Operator" or_____

Fire Department: Dial "Operator" or_____

Special Information

Bedtime _____

Meal (or snack) time _____

TV rules for children _____

Other Things Your Baby-sitter Should Know:

Names (and nicknames) of children
Sleeping arrangements
Where clothing and special equipment are kept
Favorite stories, games, and activities
Where the children play
Special habits or problems of children
Sitter's privileges (TV, radio, refrigerator)

BACKACHE   Backache can occur in a variety of conditions. It is a fairly common complaint during "flu," menstruation, acute kidney inflammations, arthritis; in some elderly individuals it is caused by shrinkage and collapse of the vertebrae due to loss of calcium. By far and away, however, the most common cause is acute and chronic stress-and-strain on the muscles and ligaments supporting the spine. Pain is most commonly experienced low in the back, either in the small of the back or in the bony region just below it (the sacroiliac region). In acute low backache severe pain may come on in seconds. The sufferer often states that he reached over to pick up something, experienced a stabbing pain in the back region, and found himself so doubled up by pain as to be unable to straighten up. A backache of this sort may be utterly incapacitating and require narcotics for relief of pain. The patient may have to be helped into bed and kept there for several days. Attempts to turn in bed may be most painful. The victim usually finds a comfortable position by trial and error. This is frequently flat on the back with a pillow underneath the knees.

Treatment. Heat from a heating pad, aspirin, and similar pain-killers—and occasionally cortisone-type drugs—may help to relieve the pain. (There are some patients who experience a few such attacks of acute sacroiliac pain at widely spread intervals throughout their lifetime.)

▶ **Chronic Low Backaches**   These may come on after a bout of acute sacroiliac strain, or may develop in a slow and progressive fashion until finally the person realizes he is having backaches a good deal of the time. Such backache is usually described as dull, persistent, and made worse under such circumstances as prolonged standing, driving, slumping in a chair, or (at times) on arising in the morning. Occasionally a single factor, such as a sagging mattress or a strain or position at work, can be identified as the cause; with correction of such a factor the backache disappears. More often, however, the patient finds that the backaches are frequent and recurrent, and that special efforts seem to be needed to help them. Among the measures that are useful are:

1. A firm mattress is generally desirable. Particularly if the pain comes on in the morning on arising, an inadequate bed

should be suspected as a major contributing factor. It may be necessary to put a bed board between mattress and box spring.

2. Attention should be directed to avoiding positions which strain the back. Chairs should have a good back support; most chairs are too deep and the victim of backache will need a pillow for adequate support. A sitting position in which the knees are at a somewhat higher level than the lower back or hips may be the most relaxing. This may be achieved by having low footstools available both at home and at work. The basic principle is to avoid positions which accentuate arching of the back.

3. Systematic daily exercises.

▶ **Exercises for Backache** Victims of chronic low backache find that exercise is the most effective therapy for their condition. Exercises should be done once or twice a day, either on a firm bed or on the floor. Among useful exercises are:

1. Lying flat on the back, raise both legs off the floor to a vertical position and slowly return to starting point.

2. In the same position, bring the legs up and over as far as possible (which will require lifting the lower back off the supporting surface).

3. Starting flat on the back, raise up the trunk, bringing arms forward until the fingertips reach the ankles.

4. "Kissing the knees:" Starting flat on the back, come up to a sitting position, at the same time drawing up the knees, thus bringing the face up to the knees.

5. From a standing position—with knees slightly bent, not with straight knees—bend the trunk, bringing arms down to ankles or toes, then return to starting position.

6. With the hands supported by top of a table or bureau and knees slightly bent—slowly do a few knee bends, then return to original position.

All these exercises can be done in sequence, with brief rest periods between them. The average sedentary person may be able to do only a few to begin with, but should be able to work up to ten to fifteen each within a period of a few weeks. In addition to their tonic and trimming effect, exercises may cause mild backaches to disappear. Although some backaches may be relieved by special belts and girdles, such devices in some cases may weaken rather than strengthen the important supporting muscles of the back and abdomen. Properly exercised and developed muscles are a better support.

BALDNESS   Baldness refers to any form of hair loss, temporary or longer lasting, in which, because of the thinning of hair, the underlying scalp becomes more readily visible. The most common form of baldness is hereditary, sex-linked, and is found in men; this form is inherited through the mother and passed on to the son. (It does not occur in women even when they carry and transmit the characteristic.) Being a female (with the accompanying female hormones) protects against this form of baldness, while being a male with male hormones predisposes. Thus a woman whose brothers are bald may pass the characteristic on to her own son even though her husband, the father of the boy, has a good head of hair. The extent of hair loss in sex-linked baldness is variable, as is also the age at which it becomes obvious. There is no treatment of significant value for this form of baldness in men, although many ingenious approaches (including the rubbing-in of female sex hormones) have been tried.

There are temporary states of hair loss in women which may unnecessarily trouble them because of the fear of significant baldness; such women may be reassured that this will not occur. Such hair loss may be seen following pregnancy, some women complaining that hair is "coming out by the handful." This form of hair loss is completely compensated for in the ensuing months.

Similar states of temporary hair loss may be seen following feverish illnesses, of which typhoid fever was once a prime example. It may be seen after some of the more common infectious diseases. Some glandular disorders may lead to noticeable hair loss; these include certain disorders of the adrenal glands and, perhaps somewhat more commonly, over- and under-function of the thyroid gland. With proper diagnosis and treatment for these conditions, however, regrowth of hair can be anticipated. Cracking and splitting of the hairs and increased shedding may occur because of some procedures applied to the hair. "Ponytails" and other styling procedures which pull unnecessarily on the hair may do this and are best avoided.

► **Alopecia Areata** A rather peculiar form of baldness seen in both sexes has been termed alopecia areata. In this disorder a circular patch of scalp loses hair. The area involved seldom exceeds the size of a quarter. After a period of some weeks or months, a regrowth of hair will occur in the bald patch. The cause of this disorder and the reason for its peculiar localization is unknown; it sometimes seems related to nervous stresses and is seen more frequently in tense, hypersensitive persons.

In elderly women, as well as in elderly men, some degree of thinning-out of the hair is generally observed. It occurs also with body hair, such as pubic and armpit hair. A somewhat similar process is being observed more frequently in a relatively small percentage of middle-aged women, no particular agent or hormonal disturbance seemingly being involved. This pattern of hair thinning in middle age seems to have arisen only in the past two decades and is still under investigation. In no way does it resemble the kinds of baldness seen in men. Women exhibiting this condition can at least be told that it is not unrestrainedly progressive; currently, hormones and other agents are being evaluated in its treatment. For practical purposes, the average woman with an average head of hair can be reasonably certain that she will keep it indefinitely, and whatever episodes of hair loss she may encounter will always be temporary ones.

BEHAVIOR AND EMOTIONS

► **Emotions in Childhood** The development of emotions or feelings begins in infancy. This refers to positive emotions (pleasure, happiness, contentment, love, etc.) as well as negative emotions (fear, anger, anxiety, depression, unhappiness, etc.). The infant is born helpless and depends for the satisfaction of his needs entirely on his mother and father. He is born into the world with certain hereditary and temperamental qualities. The development of his emotions will depend upon the nature of the interaction between him and the person who supplies his needs, usually the mother.

Inconsistent attention, stimulating or threatening behavior, punishment and hostility will give the child a sense of fear and mistrust of his environment. Sensitive mothering, with reasonable satisfaction of the emotional needs of infancy, will establish a sense of basic trust in the environment. The mother, as the recipient of signals of need from the child, has a responsibility in taking care of those needs. Her failure to do so produces in the infant feelings of anger, helplessness, insecurity, futility, and even despair. The groundwork of stable emotional development occurs during the first six to eight months of life. Overwhelming anxiety or trauma during this period can severely maim the emotional development of the child.

If a child is treated with tolerance, he learns to be patient.
If he lives with encouragement, he learns to be confident.
If he lives with praise, he learns to be appreciative.
If he lives with recognition, he learns that it is good to have a goal.
If he lives with honesty, he learns what truth is.
If he lives with fairness, he learns justice.
If he lives with security, he learns to have faith in himself and those about him.
If he lives with acceptance, he learns to love.
If he lives with friendliness, he learns the world is a nice place in which to live.
However, if he lives with criticism, he learns to condemn.
If he lives with hostility, he learns to fight.
If he lives with jealousy, he learns to feel guilty.
And if he lives with fear, he learns to be apprehensive.

The emotional climate which a child experiences in his home, school, and outer world molds his development.

▶ **Behavior Disturbances in Children**   Child behavior reflects temperament, organic problems, and social situations. Experimental evidence based on studies of children's individual primary reaction patterns, has shown what we all have more or less known for many years, namely, that different children respond to parental care practices in different ways. For instance, children may respond differently to the *same* approach on the part of the *same* parent regarding feeding, sleeping, toilet training, or general discipline. Each child seems to have a characteristic way of responding to new situations, and this response appears consistently time and again, even in more complex situations as he gets older.

Individual temperament, which consists of a number of primary reaction patterns, is one of the very important factors in the development of behavior disturbances between child and parent. A short description of some of the most important primary reaction patterns will help to clarify this concept.

1. *Adaptive and non-adaptive behavior* refers to the ability of the child to adapt to new situations and the ease with which he responds if the situation is repeated.

2. *Approach-withdrawal* refers to responses to anything new, such as foods, toys, people. Some children will approach immediately and make contact, whereas some will always be hesitant or withdrawn and have great difficulty in making contact with people and objects.

3. *Intensity* refers to the quality of a child's response to tension, hunger, new foods, attempts to discipline or restrain, dress, diapers, etc. This may be mild or extremely intense in its nature and is important in the overall picture of a child's response to various new training problems. If a child is a high intensity reactor and so is his mother, it is almost inevitable that temper tantrums and behavior disorders will occur. If the child is a mild reactor and the mother an intense person, this may still result in interpersonal difficulties. However, if both are mild reactors, presumably there is going to be less friction.

4. *Distractibility and persistence* refer to the ease with which a child can be diverted from what he is doing to doing something else. A child who is very easily distracted is going to be difficult to train. He will not be able to pay attention long enough to absorb commands. He will also probably have learning difficulties.

5. *Positive and negative moods* represent expressions of pleasure, pain, friendliness, unfriendliness, joy, and crying. A child with a high degree of negative mood responses is going to be less agreeable than a child whose responses are generally positive.

▶ **Behavior Problems, Causes of** It is important to differentiate behavior problems in children who have real organic brain damage (See BRAIN DISORDERS) and those whose temperament and ability to respond to training procedures reflect struggles with the way their parents are handling them. Disturbed functioning may represent a distortion of the characteristics of primary temperament, so that the parents respond with growing annoyance and pressure to the demonstration of the child's initial way of responding. In turn, the child's continu-

30

ing negative responses arouse parental hostility, and this leads to constant fights and recriminations within the family.

The importance and the understanding of individuality in psychological functioning cannot be overestimated. It takes sensitivity, tact, and observation for parents to see in what way their child will best respond. Usually, gentle persuasion, soft tones, and firm discipline within the framework of love and kindness will get the best results. Many behavior problems are secondary to primary disturbances, such as nightmares which result after prolonged hospitalization, or feeding problems which are secondary to prolonged illness, etc. It is necessary to have expert pediatric or psychiatric advice in cases of emotional disturbances in children.

Social situations may also create behavior disturbances in children. As children observe adults and their own friends and have a wider sampling of people to imitate, they often start imitating the disturbed behavior of classmates or of characters they see on television, in the movies, etc. They may read certain things and become influenced by them. As they grow older, various fads, customs, and social mores become standards on which they base their behavior. Children coming from one culture to another may show varieties of behavior patterns which they did not show in their original country. Gang warfare on city streets is certainly not attributable to parents but is a social phenomenon which children, unfortunately, imitate. Children who have been inadequately supervised and improperly disciplined are likely to develop serious behavior problems. Correction of severe behavior disorders of either children or adults usually requires the services of a qualified psychiatrist.

▶ **Discipline** Discipline is a matter of teaching limits to one's child. It is the process of giving the child with no life experience the benefit of the adult's experience. Discipline teaches children to set limits on their impulsive behavior, to value the rights of others, and to learn the general rules of behavior, in order to be socially accepted.

Children *require* limits. They lack a knowledge of what is good and bad for them, nor can they see far enough ahead to develop the qualities of character and internal discipline which will be necessary for their later performance as adults. Self-restraint, limitation of activities, postponement of gratification for further or future rewards are important tasks for a

31

child to learn. He has to be able to realize that breaking the rules of discipline will bring some kind of punishment, even if it is only a rebuke or an angry scolding.

Parents who continually say "no" to a child in a tone of voice which indicates contempt, anger, or scorn will soon destroy the effectiveness of this as a method of discipline. Treating a child with consideration and kindness, asking "Please do this for me," or *requesting* certain behavior is much more agreeable to anyone (including a child) than a harsh and angry command.

One of the most important aspects of obedience is the maintaining of *consistent standards of behavior* and the *maintaining of a uniform standard between both parents.* If a mother forbids something and the child says, "I'll ask father," and the father permits it, this child will soon be playing one parent off against the other in an attempt to dominate and get his own way. If the parents stick together, are firm in agreeing on methods of discipline and decisions regarding behavior, the child will have no alternative but to obey, even if unwillingly.

When repeated training and discipline take effect, the child learns inner control, so that he can begin to discipline himself in life situations and get along without the constant help of his parents. Discipline involves guidance, assistance, acceptance, and permitting growth while imposing limits on unacceptable behavior. His self-discipline will enhance his self-esteem and give him confidence in life. But remember, the language of love and authority can be the same.

▶ **Temper Tantrums** Temper tantrums are a form of manipulative behavior on the part of a child, characterized by screaming, kicking, breath-holding, and extreme agitation. This response is often seen in infants or very young children when they are frustrated or refused something they badly want. They may become angry or jealous and may use this method to blackmail parents into giving in to them. It is a fairly common behavior reaction in children from one to four. Temper tantrums which occur in older age groups (children of eight, nine, or adolescents) are a more serious behavior disorder and will require different treatment.

If a temper tantrum is met with indifference and nonchalance, the child will soon observe that kicking and screaming serve no good purpose and are self-defeating procedures. If a child is given what he wishes because the parents become intimidated, he will learn that he can do this whenever he wishes to get his way. It is a very bad emotional habit to encourage. It is not usually necessary to punish the child who has temper tantrums. Just refusing to acknowledge him and handling the situation with calm and firm tolerance is probably the best procedure.

Impulse control and its mastery are a requirement of normal emotional development. Temper tantrums may sometimes occur in neurologically damaged or defective children because of inability to control their impulses. In these cases it may be necessary to treat them with medication and sedation.

▶ **Neurosis in Childhood** Neuroses and mental disturbances begin to exist in childhood. The manner in which a child deals with his environment and with his relations to parents and other significant persons determines many of the characteristics of his behavior in later life.

Neurotic character disorders are characterized by very fixed and pervading attitudes in which the child has a distorted impression of other people's attitudes, behavior and motives. A child may think that every person he meets is going to behave in a threatening or destructive manner toward him and adopt a character pattern of defensive hostility, aggression, or withdrawal. If this expectation of threatening behavior becomes inflexible, the child will react to every person in his environment in exactly the same abnormal manner.

In order to prevent serious adult character neuroses, children with these behavior disorders should be treated by a child psychiatrist or a psychologist early in the disturbance. Otherwise the disorder becomes magnified, ingrained into the personality, and is extremely difficult, if not impossible, to erase later in life.

Phobias and anxiety reactions in children may be real or may be irrational. A child may become frightened of the water after having a near-drowning experience, but usually the reaction to this, if he develops normally, should be gradual restoration of confidence in his ability to go into the water and learn how to swim. A child may be frightened by a horse or a dog, but later on becomes adjusted to the idea that not all dogs or horses are dangerous. If this ability to change fails to develop, various phobias and fears may appear, with many of the more irrational ones, which are incomprehensible and baffling to parents, representing substitutions for deeper-hidden fears. These require unraveling by a qualified child psychiatrist.

Bed-wetting (Enuresis) Bed-wetting is involuntary urination during sleep or in daytime. It may be caused by infections or abnormalities of the urinary system. It may be caused by inability of the bladder to hold enough fluid. It is usually only a problem if it persists beyond the age of three or four and if its occurrence is frequent.

Most children who can develop speech have the ability to hold urine long enough to notify their parents when they have to urinate. Bed-wetting may sometimes represent a regression to a previous immature state during periods of emotional stress or upset. Some cases of bed-wetting are purely psychological, and it will take a trained physician to determine whether this is so. Even if it is psychological, however, it is usually not conscious or voluntary, so that the child is actually unable to control it. He may have to be retrained and reconditioned. There are some devices available for conditioning children. They generally involve a bell which rings as the child starts to urinate. Feeding of small amounts of salty foods at bedtime, and limiting fluids after 6 p.m., may help to control night bed-wetting. It is not advisable to humiliate or punish children for this difficulty. Such an approach may simply aggravate the condition.

Nail-biting (Onychophagy) This is a common sign of nervousness, tension, excitement, or worry in a child. It may indicate fear and anxiety or may be an expression of repressed anger.

Treatment is directed to allaying the fear, anxiety, or nervousness and to trying to provide more stable emotional support for the child. Punishment for this habit is usually useless and often only aggravates the condition. Putting ill-tasting medicine on the nails and shaming or punishing the child usually intensifies nail-biting. A child who bites his nails out of boredom or lack of interests should be directed toward some meaningful activity to keep his hands occupied.

Nightmares (Night Terrors) Nightmares, night terrors, and bad dreams occur in children who may be restless, emotionally upset, neurotic, or suffering from some mild illness. Many of

34

these episodes represent dreams of anxiety, psychic conflict, and fears. They may reflect a frightening or traumatic situation which the child has experienced during the day. He may relive these fearful experiences at night and wake with fears and anxiety. Sometimes frightening things seen on television or in movies may distress the child and he will dream about them. They may represent fear resulting from a disturbed relationship with or between the parents. They may also represent displacements of anxiety in the form of phobic fears.

During an attack of night terrors, the child suddenly wakes up, cries out or screams, trembling and perspiring. He may be incoherent and not understand what has frightened him. He may or may not remember the occurrence in the morning.

The immediate treatment of a frightening dream is to try to reassure the child, comfort him, and try to get him back to sleep. If the child is old enough to comprehend, he can be told it was "only a bad dream." Since many children dream about frightening experiences (such as watching horror shows), stimulating television or movie programs should be avoided by these sensitive children. Any child who persistently has nightmares or night terrors should be evaluated by a psychiatrist to determine whether there is an emotional disorder present. A complete psychological and psychiatric examination is often required.

▶ **Oedipus Complex and Electra Complex** A complex is a group of associated ideas (which may be partly unconscious) that have strong emotional overtones. They may significantly influence attitudes and associations.

The Oedipus complex, first described by Sigmund Freud, refers to the attachment of the male child for his parent of the opposite sex accompanied by feelings of envy and aggression toward the parent of his own sex. Attitudes arising during critical phases of infantile emotional development and largely repressed (made unconscious) because of fear of punishment by the parent of the same sex are responsible for the complex. Originally the term was used only in relation to male children. A parallel type of complex has long been recognized as existing in girls and is called the Electra complex. Both of these terms are derived from Greek mythology.

Inadequate mastery of the emotions during the "oedipal" period results in prolonged (unconscious) emotional attachments and persistence of emotional disorders resulting in neurosis.

▶ **Extroversion and Introversion** *Extroversion* is the name given to a personality type whose attention and energies are directed outward from the self, as opposed to introversion, in which interest is directed primarily toward one's own self. In the latter condition there is a reduction of interest in the outside world. Naturally, there are gradations and degrees of both personality types, and there are times in the life of any person when he may become more introverted than he normally is (states of grief, sadness, depression). The degree to which these states become exaggerated and, therefore, pathological is a criterion for normal or abnormal mental states.

▶ **Depression** Depression is one of the most universal of all human emotions. No one can expect to go through life without experiencing depressions. A depression brought about by sad events, failures, or financial reverses (and thus one which is entirely understandable) is sometimes referred to as a reactive depression. It is not always possible to identify the causes of depressions, however. Some seem to arise almost spontaneously from within; to put it another way, the events that trigger them seem to be insufficient causes. Some of the depressions that are seen in middle-aged individuals fall into this category and are sometimes referred to as endogenous depressions.

Some of the cyclic depressions to which women may be subject are essentially transitory. Their widespread occurrence suggests that they may depend on hormonal or other processes going on within the system. Thus the premenstrual tension and depression which affect a considerable number of women have been related to hormones with fluid-retaining properties. These psychic complaints appear with, and seem to be more marked in women who complain of considerable bloating and swelling. The depression often ends quite promptly with the onset of menstruation, at which time there is an abrupt drop-off in the hormones responsible.

▶ **Depressive Reactions** Depressive reactions can occur under other circumstances than the reproductive ones, such as menstruation and delivery. Some individuals (for reasons that often become clear only when their whole life history is reviewed) may be subject to recurrent bouts of depression. There

36

are some families in which several members may from time to time be afflicted with fairly severe depressions. Some of these troublesome depressions are associated with feelings of inferiority, self-blame, and self-attack, deep feelings of pessimism about life and the desirability of living, etc. Depressive reactions of this sort can be brought about by any of a great number of major events and having a baby is only one of them.

Drugs may be helpful in at least alleviating such depressive states, but when there is a pattern of recurrent depressions some form of psychotherapy may well be the answer and provide a more permanent and superior solution. The aim in psychotherapy is for the patient to find out why he or she has feelings of inadequacy, poor self-esteem, convictions of unworthiness, and other similar ideas which often form the basis for depression. Psychotherapy may take time and is frequently quite expensive, nevertheless there are circumstances in which it is wise to consider it, or at least discuss the possibility of such treatment with a physician.

▶ **Psychopathic Personality** This refers to a child or adult who is unable to be disciplined, who performs impulsive antisocial acts without any understanding of the feelings of others, and without any qualms regarding his disturbed behavior. It also refers to a person *who has never been taught limits:* that he sometimes should delay or postpone gratification, that a sense of guilt should follow wrongdoing. It implies the inability to develop a "conscience" or a sense of self-limitation. It implies the inability to see reality properly or to learn from experience or disaster. A child who is habitually cruel, destructive, intolerant of the feelings of others, shows characteristics of this disorder. These children urgently require treatment; otherwise they will grow up to become serious delinquent and criminal problems.

Most behavior problems which begin in childhood and continue untreated into adolescence will show up as adolescent character disorders. Personality traits may carry over, show feelings of self-contempt and unworthiness, attitudes of arrogance and contempt, hostility and exploitation. Or on the other hand, they may show continued dependency and inability to rely on the self. Children may also show attitudes of excessive ingratiation or an attempt to please others, which is equally abnormal since it does not show an adequate concern for one's self as an individual.

The aim of raising children is to raise mature, independent, functioning adults. The mentally healthy person can deal with reality even at its worst, find satisfaction in struggle (including adversity which can be turned into achievement). The mentally healthy person is relatively free from tensions and anxieties, relates consistently to others with mutual satisfaction and helpfulness. He accepts present frustration in the hopes of future gains, profits from experience, and can direct and divert hostile feelings into creative or constructive outlets. Finally, he has the capacity to love, the most essential quality of human behavior.

▶ **Psychosis in Children** This indicates a state of clinical "insanity" which may occur in a child who has normal capacity but has been so traumatized, so badly treated and handled in childhood, that he becomes quite abnormal. Some of these children are called schizophrenic. Psychoses in children also refer to the behavior of children who have brain disturbances and are damaged. Their behavior is fragmented, irrational, hyperactive, and very disordered—but on the basis of an organic condition. Some children who are mentally defective or retarded may also show behavior disturbances which are classified as psychotic. (See also BRAIN DISORDERS.)

▶ **Psychotherapy** Psychotherapy is a form of medical treatment for emotional and mental illness which attempts to uncover the meanings and the origins of the disorder. Unlike other procedures (which may also be useful)—such as the taking of drugs, changes in the environment, or electroconvulsive treatment—most psychotherapy involves a series of discussions between patient and doctor. Generally the patient discusses his symptoms, his feelings, and many aspects of his personal development. From time to time the psychotherapist may organize and interpret this material in a new and meaningful way. By this process the patient develops insight and, as a result of the deepened understanding he gains of himself, many behavioral changes can follow. One of the key concepts that may emerge is the patient's understanding of anxiety. It is anxiety experienced early in life which can lead to later difficulties in a person's behavior—whether in the family, at work, or in the sexual or social areas.

For adults, the most sophisticated form of psychotherapy is known as analysis. In the course of this, the patient speaks out freely, letting his thoughts come out as they may and using dreams or daily events as points of departure. This technique is known as free association and can lead to surprising insights.

Although with adults it is possible to interchange ideas through talk, this may not be the case with a young child, for whom a type of treatment is used known as "play therapy." In one form of play therapy, a large number of dolls which can be perceived as parents, children, and pets are made available to the child, and his behavior with them is studied. A skilled child therapist will make available to the child appropriate toys and games to reveal his disturbance. Psychotherapy has been criticized from time to time as being an imperfect instrument; but imperfect or not, it is at present the only instrument available for the treatment of some emotional difficulties in children as well as adults.

BIRTH CONTROL   Birth control refers to any of those procedures which will diminish or do away with the probability of pregnancy; it is also known as family planning and contraception. Besides the inadequate methods, such as *coitus interruptus,* and tap-water douche, that have been employed, the more effective or better known ones are the following:

1. *Birth-control pills.* Their effectiveness is approximately 100 per cent. Many kinds are dispensed in a special package containing 20 pills. Counting the first day of menstruation as day 1 of the cycle, the pill is taken on the morning of day 5 and every morning thereafter through day 25. Within a few days of stopping—roughly therefore around day 28—menstruation occurs. Again one waits till day 5 and repeats the daily taking of the pill. The pills work by preventing the growth and release of the egg from the ovary, so that a woman remains infertile throughout her cycle. Once the pills are stopped, the possibility of pregnancy promptly recurs; thus it is necessary for the pill to be taken daily. Occasionally pink staining may occur while taking the pills; this may necessitate a temporary increase in the amount taken. Other difficulties are occasional symptoms of nausea or bloating. An increased amount of clotting in the veins was reported for the first pill in use. Since then, a reduction in dose and newer combina-

tions have been made available, and original difficulties may now be reduced.

2. *Diaphragm.* This is a rubber dome mounted on a flexible rubber-covered metal circle. When properly inserted, it fits into the upper portion of the vagina, covering the opening to the uterus (the cervix). Usually a special sperm-killing jelly or cream is used to seal the edges of the diaphragm.

3. *Condom.* Sometimes referred to as "a rubber," this is a device worn by the male. It is convenient, and widely used.

4. *Foams and jellies.* These are sperm-killing materials injected or placed within the vagina just before intercourse. They rapidly immobilize and kill the sperm. They are fairly effective, generally non-irritating, and lessen the need for the fitting or insertion of a diaphragm.

5. *Rhythm method.* Sometimes also referred to as the "safe period."

▶ **"Safe Period" (Rhythm System)** The "safe period" is the time in a woman's menstrual cycle when she cannot become pregnant. In the average woman it generally refers to a few days after the end of menstruation and to a period of about a week-and-a-half before the expected onset of her next menstruation. A knowledge of the safe cycle is basic to the rhythm method of birth control. It is based upon the following considerations:

1. An egg is released (ovulation) from a woman's ovary only once during a menstrual cycle.

2. The egg can be fertilized by the sperm of the male only during about twenty-four hours after its release. After that time the egg undergoes degenerative changes and can no longer initiate a pregnancy.

3. Although the sperm supplied by the male can live for a somewhat longer period within the female reproductive tract, they probably cannot fertilize the egg more than two or three days after their release.

4. If one could time the ovulation exactly, and if no sperm were supplied for approximately three days before, and for a day or two afterwards, pregnancy could not occur. The time in the cycle just before and just after the release of the egg is the time of highest fertility in a woman; other parts of the menstrual cycle would therefore be "safe"

The difficulty arising with this approach is that the menstrual cycle is subject to some fluctuation. Even very regular women find, when they start charting their cycle on the calendar, that it fluctuates either way by several days. It is also known that ovulation may occur somewhat earlier in some cycles and be somewhat later in other cycles, although most ovulations in a woman with a twenty-eight-day cycle tend to occur around days 12, 13, and 14 of the cycle (day 1 of the cycle is the first day of menstruation).

To take into account the different menstrual cycles the following has been proposed. A woman should keep track of the length of her menstrual cycles for approximately a year. By subtracting 18 from her shortest cycle and 11 from her longest cycle she can calculate the time of her highest fertility. Intercourse without contraception during this time would be the most likely to result in pregnancy. Furthermore, it cannot be applied to a woman whose cycles fluctuate a good deal—if one menstrual cycle is twenty-three days and another thirty-three days the method will not be reliable.

RHYTHM THEORY OF BIRTH CONTROL

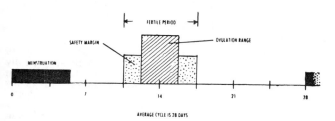

AVERAGE CYCLE IS 28 DAYS

BIRTHMARKS, FRECKLES, AND MOLES

▶ **Angioma** Angiomas are small skin lesions characterized by an elevated red area having small dilated capillaries radiating from it like a spider's legs. These are called *spider nevi*. They are usually birthmarks and frequently disappear. If they persist, they may be treated with electrolysis or electrocautery.

▶ **Cavernous Angioma** This is the most common birthmark.

41

It is more deep-seated than the others and is sometimes called a strawberry angioma because of its resemblance to a strawberry. It varies in size. The treatment is usually with sclerosing agents which are injected at intervals into the lesion until it disappears. Carbon dioxide snow is also used to shrink the involved vessels. Some types which are very extensive may require surgical removal.

► **Port-wine Mark** This is a more extensive birthmark, involving larger areas of the skin. The port-wine discoloration of the skin is caused by a network of fine capillaries. It becomes redder if the child cries or strains. Most of these marks are somewhat disfiguring when they appear on the face. There are waterproof cosmetics available at a drug store which cover marks temporarily.

► **Freckles** Freckles are flat, vari-colored, pigmented areas of the skin. Freckling is usually hereditary and appears in darkly pigmented as well as light-skinned peoples. Sunlight causes freckles to increase. They are harmless. However, one form, which is blue-black in color and is slightly raised, may be pre-malignant. This form is called a melanoma. It is dangerous to remove these lesions, as they may spread to other areas of the body. Surgical removal requires wide excision. Doctors with skill and experience should be consulted regarding removal of any freckle.

► **Moles** Few, if any of us, are lacking in at least a small number of moles, and in some individuals there are literally hundreds of them. Most are small, perhaps ¼-½ inch in length, and are to be found almost anywhere on the skin. They are mostly tan, brown or blue-black in color, often slightly elevated, and may bear a few hairs. It is not practical to remove most moles, nor is it necessary. If a mole is considered to be a cosmetic problem the doctor can easily remove it, often by as simple a procedure as cauterizing. This will, of course, result in a small scar. In general moles are to be regarded as harmless.

An exceedingly rare tumor related to moles is known as a melanoma. Melanomas may arise in a pre-existent type of mole (known as the junctional nevus) which appears as a generally flat, blue to black, hairless pigment spot in the skin. Some also appear to arise in apparently normal skin without a preceding nevus. Melanomas occur most often on the hands, feet or genitals. Any mole that enlarges, becomes darker or develops nearby new pigment spots, ulcerates or bleeds should be called to the doctor's attention.

None of these moles is in any way related to the patchy pigmentation of the skin that occurs in some pregnancies. This is most marked on the face and resembles patches of tan. It is sometimes so extensive as to be called "the mask of pregnancy." It is probably due to a pigment-controlling secretion from the pituitary gland. The pigmentation recedes after the delivery.

BITES, ANIMAL, INSECT AND SNAKE

▶ **Animal Bites** Most animal bites present no special problems of infection, with a few exceptions. The risk of infection is cut further if one permits some bleeding from the wound or even encourages bleeding with slight pressure, as in the case of puncture wounds produced by a cat. One may then wash the wound with soap and water which may be all the first-aid procedures that are needed. If there is free bleeding, such as may occur from a dog-inflicted laceration, a clean compress can be applied and firm pressure maintained. If the skin is not penetrated by a bite, there need be no further concern. This can be the case when a dog bites through heavy clothing, or in the relatively uncommon bites from a horse; both may produce a bruising injury only, for which application of an ice bag may be useful in cutting down swelling and bleeding within the skin. Very rarely, and only after the passage of some weeks, scratches or bites from cats may produce fever and swelling of the nearby lymph glands. This is known as cat-scratch fever. Rabies following a dog bite is even rarer. However, if the dog is a stray, is known not to have been immunized, behaves peculiarly, or runs about snapping and biting aimlessly, it should be captured and turned over to the authorities for further examination. If this is not done and a question arises as to whether or not the dog might have been rabid, it may become necessary to give the bite victim a course of special injections known as the Pasteur treatment.

▶ **Insect Bites** *Bites of mosquitoes and gnats* will produce immediate itching, and itching may recur thereafter for one or more days. They are generally disregarded. However, a paste of soda bicarbonate or a pledget of cotton dipped in household ammonia diluted with three parts of water may be dabbed on the bite. Calamine lotion may be applied for recurrent itching.

Bee bites can be treated by removal of the stinger with a forceps or tweezer, followed by local application of ice, then by calamine lotion or a paste of bicarbonate of soda. Bee bites can be dangerous and even fatal to sensitive individuals. Indications of such sensitivity are unusual local swelling, and marked general reactions such as weakness, faintness or collapse. If any such unusual reactions do occur with a child or adult, hypersensitivity exists and any further exposure to bee bites can be most hazardous. Extracts for producing desensitization are available and should be used in such cases. Otherwise strict avoidance of the countryside and areas where bee bites can occur is necessary. If exposure is unavoidable and undue sensitivity may still be present, tablets to be placed under the tongue (Isuprel®) or an adrenalin inhaler such as is used by asthmatics should be carried on the person. The fact is that there are more fatalities from bee bite than from snakebite or any other kind of animal bite.

A few *spider bites* present special threats: the black widow spider, which is recognizable by the orange hourglass figure on its abdomen, injects a toxin which can produce serious general reactions including painful contractions of all muscles and collapse. It is found mostly in the southern United States. The brown recluse spider is found most commonly in the southwestern United States, most often in the cellars and basements of buildings. It does not attack unless disturbed. Its bite can produce a marked local breakdown of the skin as well as general reactions.

Scorpion bites also lead to an introduction of a toxin under the skin. They are not likely to be serious except in very small children. First aid for all of these bites may consist of tying a tourniquet above the site of the bite, much as for snakebite, and the application of ice to the area of bite. The patient should be taken to any nearby doctor's office or medical facility.

▶ **Snakebites** Most United States snakes are harmless. Poisonous snakes have fangs—specialized teeth through which a poison can be injected under the skin as with a hypodermic needle. The bite is characteristically two needle-like puncture

44

wounds side by side. The only four poisonous snakes in the United States are the rattlesnake, the cottonmouth moccasin, the copperhead, and the coral snake. First aid for their bites includes the following:

1. *Immediately apply a tourniquet* some inches above the wound at a level where the soft tissues can be compressed; tighten the tourniquet to a point where the veins swell up and the skin becomes flushed.

2. With a sharp razor blade or knife *make an X-shaped incision* over each of the fang marks. The cut can be up to one quarter of an inch deep. Avoid prominent skin vessels such as veins, or any tendons.

3. *Suck out the venom,* which will be mixed with blood. Spit it out from time to time but keep sucking as strongly as possible for at least an hour. If there are no open cuts in the mouth the venom is harmless, and it is equally harmless if swallowed.

4. *Have the victim lie down* and keep the suction going while he is being taken to a hospital or the doctor's office.

5. A snakebite kit may well be kept in the car or with camping equipment if one is going into areas where poisonous snakes are known to exist.

BLADDER DISORDERS

▶ **Cystitis** The most common disorder affecting the bladder is an inflammation termed cystitis. It is a good deal more common in women than in men. Cystitis produces an entire set of uncomfortable symptoms, among which are:

1. *Frequent desire to urinate.* Although the bladder feels as though it is full, so that the desire to urinate may be quite urgent, only small amounts of urine are passed; nonetheless the patient may find it necessary to go to the bathroom every few minutes throughout the day.

2. Frequent complaint of *painful urination.* This is often described as a burning pain.

3. Sometimes, because of painful spasm around the bladder opening, it is *difficult to start urination,* and the urine may come in weak, dribbling fashion.

4. Not uncommonly, there is *some bleeding* associated with cystitis. It is seldom more than enough to color the urine in

an obvious fashion and is sometimes mistaken for vaginal bleeding.

Treatment. Fortunately, these distressing symptoms will generally respond within a day or so to the administration of antibiotic or sulfa drugs. In fact, the symptoms often improve markedly, even though some pus and bacteria can still be found in the urine. Cystitis is generally treated for a matter of some days, or even longer; the urine should be checked, not only when treatment is discontinued but also at some intervals thereafter. The aim is to avoid any lurking, low-grade, or chronic infection which can go unnoticed but may serve as a source of reinfection and flare-up of cystitis later. Most cases of cystitis, if untreated, tend to get progressively worse. There is very often an ascending spread of the infection to the kidneys, at which point symptoms such as chills and fever often occur.

▶ **Cystocele** This is the medical term for a sagging of the bladder produced by a relaxation of the tissues supporting it. It is limited to women who have been pregnant and is seen as an occasional sequel to pregnancy and delivery. Only a small minority of mothers, however, develop cystocele of any consequence, and mild degrees of cystocele can be disregarded.

A large cystocele is detected easily enough by inspection. The patient is told to bear down as though she were having a bowel movement. The increased pressure within the abdomen will push the sagging bladder down into the upper wall of the vagina, thus producing a bulge at the vaginal opening. It is this anatomical fact that leads to the difficulties of cystocele, for it may be difficult or impossible to evacuate the bladder completely. This alone may lead to frequency of urination. It is also a general fact that infection is likely to occur whenever the bladder cannot be completely emptied. Thus there may be frequent episodes of cystitis with all the discomfort that these can bring. It is sometimes possible, at least partially, to correct the difficulty produced by a cystocele by inserting a pessary into the vagina to support the bladder.

For cystocele of a degree that produces frequent symptoms or infections, surgery is recommended. The aim is to fashion a sling of supporting tissue that will hold the bladder in a normal location. When this is done, the symptoms due to cystocele disappear.

► **Rectocele** Very often, in addition to cystocele, rectocele may be present. This is an anatomically similar condition, but in this case it is the rectum that bulges into the lower wall of the vagina. A rectocele may produce relatively few symptoms except when quite large, and is generally disregarded. However, it is possible surgically to repair a rectocele at the same time that the cystocele is repaired.

BLEEDING

► **Cuts and Lacerations** Bleeding from a large cut or laceration can be brisk if one of the larger veins or arteries is cut. The best generally applicable method for control of such bleeding is to *exert firm pressure, using a cloth compress, against the area.* In an emergency one can employ a wad of facial tissue, a handkerchief, towel, shirt, or a pillowcase suitably folded on itself so as to make the compress. Press it against the bleeding site, and if the cut is on a limb, elevate the limb, for this too diminishes bleeding. Maintain pressure for five to ten minutes. One may then lift part of the compress to judge whether the bleeding has come under control. If it has not, pressure can be maintained for a longer period or even indefinitely if necessary.

► **Nosebleed** In principle a nosebleed is treated in the same manner. Almost all nosebleeds occur from the septum, the central partition that separates the nostrils. This is made of cartilage (gristle). It has a rich blood supply, chiefly of smaller blood vessels. To control bleeding from this, grasp the fleshy portion of the nose firmly between the thumb and forefinger, and keep it compressed for five to ten minutes.

► **Pressure Points** Pressure points are places where major arteries can be directly compressed—often against a bone— thus cutting down the circulation to a limb or other part of the body. A knowledge of pressure points and their use forms part of advanced first-aid courses and requires considerable practice and training. Two such points that everyone might readily become familiar with are the brachial and femoral. The brachial artery can be felt high up on the inner surface of the arm just below the armpit. It can be recognized by its pulsation, and the vessel can be readily compressed against the unyielding arm bone alongside of it. It is the major artery

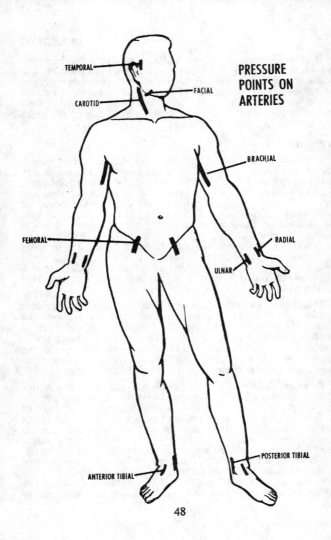

PRESSURE POINTS ON ARTERIES

TEMPORAL

FACIAL

CAROTID

BRACHIAL

FEMORAL

RADIAL

ULNAR

POSTERIOR TIBIAL

ANTERIOR TIBIAL

supplying the entire upper extremity. The corresponding artery for the entire lower extremity, the femoral artery, can be located in the crease between thigh and abdomen. The arterial pulse can be felt at about the middle of the crease, and the vessel is readily compressed against the firm tissues beneath it.

▶ **Tourniquets—Severe Bleeding** Another first-aid method occasionally needed *to control severe bleeding* is the tourniquet. A tourniquet can be improvised by tying a handkerchief, a strip of cloth, or rope of clothesline diameter (a tourniquet that is too narrow may cut into the tissues.) Next a stick, heavy pencil, or even a butter knife is placed between the skin and the encircling handkerchief. Turn this one or more times, thus tightening the encircling cloth. If the pressure is inadequate, the part of the limb below the tourniquet will turn reddish, the veins will increase in size and bleeding may actually increase. If the constricting pressure is raised above the level of the pressure in the arteries, the portion of the limb below the tourniquet turns white and bleeding should stop or markedly subside. The pressure of a tourniquet can be released (preferably by a doctor) at ten-to-fifteen-minute intervals to check on whether bleeding has stopped. Overlong use (longer than one hour or so) of a tourniquet may put the limb in jeopardy.

▶ **Internal Bleeding** There are no first-aid measures for hemorrhage of internal organs; indeed, it is not often easy to recognize it. Thus a person with a bleeding peptic ulcer may vomit blood, or pass a very black stool; sometimes he merely becomes very dizzy or faints. Large-scale internal bleeding can be recognized by weakness, pallor, rapid pulse. The patient should lie down, and no whiskey or other stimulants should be given. If there is any possibility of delay in securing a doctor, precious time is best saved by rushing the patient directly to a hospital.

▶ **Hemophilia** This is a hereditary disease occurring in males and transmitted by females. A disease of excessive and easy bleeding, it is believed to be caused by a deficiency of plasma thromboplastinogen. Formation of thrombin, needed for clot formation, is lacking, and consequently, no blood clot forms. Bleeding may be controlled by application of cold packs locally; otherwise, plasma transfusions and transfusions of antihemophiliac globulin and 50 per cent fibrinogen transfusions have been helpful. There is no cure.

49

▶ **Thrombocytopenic Purpura** This disease is characterized by small, spontaneous hemorrhages into the skin, the mucous membrane, and other tissues of the body. It occurs most often in females under the age of twelve.

Symptoms. Bleeding may be from the nose or mouth, and there may be black-and-blue marks over the surface of the body. It may be due to infection, drugs, diseases, vitamin deficiency, or no particular cause may be found for it. There is usually a lack of platelets in the peripheral blood, which produces a defect in the clotting mechanism. Since clots do not form at the torn capillaries, bleeding time is prolonged.

Treatment. Newer drugs, such as ACTH and cortisone, have been used with limited success. Occasionally, removal of the spleen is required in long-standing cases.

BLOOD, THE Two groups of cells are moved along the circulating blood. One, the red blood cells, is involved in the transfer of oxygen to the tissues and is responsible for the red color of blood; the other, the white blood cells, takes part in the body's defense, as in inflammation. There are several groups of white blood cells—lymphocytes, plasma cells, polymorphonuclear leukocytes—each with different properties and making different contributions to defense. The polymorphonuclear leukocytes, for example, are involved in acute inflammation against bacteria; thus they are the major cells found in pus.

Enumeration of blood cells, known as a *blood count,* is a routine and basic examination in medicine. A complete blood count may call for several more bits of information:

1. An estimate of hemoglobin (the essential component of the red blood cell).

2. A differential white blood cell count, in which the white blood cells are stained and the different kinds counted.

3. Occasionally, a platelet count—a count of the tiny cellular fragments, or platelets, which play an important role in blood-clotting.

The blood count is an important diagnostic clue. In anemia both the red blood cell count and the hemoglobin count fall. In leukemia, the white blood cells are abnormal and often very high in number. The white blood cell count is generally high when there is infection due to bacteria, but barely elevated and sometimes even low in many infections due to viruses. The white cells increase as an infection worsens and decrease as it subsides. In allergic disorders a special kind of white cell known as the eosinophil may be considerably increased. Changes in white cells occur in infectious mononucleosis. Low counts for all types of cells may be found in certain disorders of the spleen and bone marrow. (See also ANEMIA.)

▶ **Albumin** Albumin is an important protein manufactured in the liver, which circulates in the blood stream. Human albumin is a pale, somewhat sticky material, quite like the white of an egg. In certain disorders albumin may pass through the small blood vessels of the kidney and appear in the urine. One of the basic tests in medicine is, therefore, the test for albuminuria—the presence of albumin in urine. Here albumin may be found as a result of acute or chronic inflammation of the kidneys; as a result of the effect of high blood pressure on the kidneys, or in circulatory disorders affecting the kidneys, such as heart failure.

Some drugs and poisons may damage the kidneys sufficiently to produce albuminuria. This condition may also be due to quite innocuous causes, such as fever. In a few individuals, albumin appears in the urine when they assume the upright position, although not present when they are lying down. This is known as orthostatic albuminuria; it is of no great concern but may lead to diagnostic difficulties. One of the few threatening disorders associated with pregnancy, known as eclampsia, has various warning symptoms and findings, such as rise in blood pressure, headache, and puffiness around the eyes and elsewhere. Generally associated with these is the finding of albumin in the urine. Eclampsia illustrates one of the reasons for doing routine urinalysis during pregnancy.

One rather serious affliction of the kidneys—the nephrotic syndrome—results from various kinds of inflammations and also from advanced diabetes; large amounts of albumin are poured out into the urine and because of the loss of this important protein, marked swelling of the various tissues (edema) occurs. The major change that underlies all forms of this disorder is loss of albumin into the urine.

▶ **Gamma Globulin** Second in amount to the albumin in the circulating blood are the globulins. These are a group of diverse proteins which can be separated from one another by

51

appropriate chemical procedures. The most important one which is now commercially available is gamma globulin. It is formed by the lymphocyte-plasma cell group of the white blood cells, and is part of the body's chemical defenses against infection.

The disease-fighting globulins are sometimes referred to as *antibodies;* without antibodies it would be impossible to develop immunity, and we would be fighting the same disease battles over and over again. As it is, one successful battle may result in the production of enough antibodies to protect the individual against that organism for the rest of his life. For this reason, an adult who has had measles or hepatitis can be exposed to a child with the disease and not reacquire it. In fact, such antibodies are produced even when the disease is nipped in the bud; thus a person may be exposed to the viruses of polio, hepatitis, or mumps and overcome them without the characteristic signs of the disease, be it the paralysis of polio or the jaundice of hepatitis. These brief battles may produce relatively few symptoms beyond fever and grippal sensations, often cannot be diagnosed, but nonetheless produce immunity. Hence commercially obtained gamma globulin made from a pool derived from many individuals is a storehouse filled with all sorts of specialized weapons capable of fighting a variety of infective processes.

The value of gamma globulin is pointed up by recorded cases of a relatively rare condition known as agammaglobulinemia. Some babies are born with this condition, while some children and adults acquire it later in life. These individuals are unable to form adequate amounts of antibodies and are subject to repetition of the same illnesses, most often respiratory illnesses with bouts of pneumonia. They may also have the same contagious disease more than once and it may not be possible to immunize them successfully. Indeed, one way of diagnosing the condition is to demonstrate the inability of a child to form antitoxins to scarlet fever or diphtheria toxins. Such children, however, may be given some degree of enhanced protection against infections by repeated doses of gamma globulin.

The most common use of gamma globulin is in preventing certain infections in exposed individuals or in diminishing the severity of an illness. It is common medical procedure to give small doses of gamma globulin to all household contacts when a case of infectious hepatitis appears. In children who have been exposed to measles, a small dose of gamma globulin given at the appropriate time may diminish the severity of the measles attack, producing "modified measles." A more recent application is the administration of gamma globulin in a small dose at the time of a measles vaccination. A very mild form of measles results and the child develops immunity despite the mildness of the modified disease. It is occasionally recommended that a large dose of gamma globulin be given to individuals who are traveling into areas with a high incidence of hepatitis, such as India. The dose gives protection for a period of about six weeks and has been shown statistically to diminish the possibility of hepatitis developing. Various other claims have been made for the protective value of gamma globulin, such as an ability to cut down the number of respiratory infections in children, but they have not been verified.

BLOOD PRESSURE   Determination of blood pressure yields two measurements: the *systolic,* which measures the height of the pressure produced by the thrust of the heart; and the *diastolic,* which measures the constant "head of pressure" that exists between the beats. A blood pressure of 120 /80, for example, would record a normal systolic and a normal diastolic pressure.

Blood pressure may vary considerably in the same individual at different times in his life. It may show a rise under the influence of emotions, in cold weather, as an effect of drugs, and (sometimes) during the course of pregnancy. It may be lower in hot weather, when the person is resting or has taken sedatives, during a fainting spell, or as a result of shock. In contrast, it may also be remarkably stable from year to year.

The cutoff point at which high or low blood pressure is diagnosed is somewhat arbitrary and many people have borderline readings or may be somewhat high on one occasion and normal on another. Systolic blood pressure readings of less than 100 would be regarded as rather low for an adult; however, they are encountered in many perfectly healthy persons. In the diagnosis of high blood pressure or hypertension the diastolic blood pressure is of the greater importance. A diastolic blood pressure of 90-95 may be regarded as borderline elevation, and most doctors would agree that once it exceeds 100, high blood pressure exists. The diastolic blood pressure is more important because it represents a constant pressure to which the arteries are subjected. Thus a blood pressure reading of 130/100 might be regarded as a case of hypertension which should be treated, whereas one of 170/80 could well be regarded as normal, particularly for an elderly person, and in any case not presenting a need for treatment.

► **Hypertension (High Blood Pressure)** When levels of blood pressure significantly exceed normal, hypertension or high blood pressure is said to exist. A rise in blood pressure may occur acutely, as when a person is frightened, angry, or even as a result of the anxiety that some people are apt to experience when they go to the doctor's office. On relaxation, such a person's blood pressure may return to normal. A fairly sustained rise in blood pressure may occur throughout a pregnancy, with a return to normal soon after the delivery; this is often associated with an unusual degree of fluid retention and is thought to be due to secretions emanating from the pregnant uterus. Certain tumors of the adrenal glands known as pheochromocytomas may similarly produce secretions that raise the blood pressure, and there are many disorders of the kidney in which rises in blood pressure occur.

A great majority of cases of hypertension have no ascertainable causes of this sort and are spoken of as *essential hypertension*. Essential hypertension is found in about 20 per cent of the population and runs through some families, so that a constitutional factor seems to be involved. It is sometimes possible to identify individuals who will develop sustained hypertension later in life by abnormal rises in response to tension or to cold exposure. There are sound reasons for identifying and treating hypertension early in its course. Hypertension increases the work of the heart, the muscular wall of the left ventricle (whose contraction pumps out the blood) undergoing enlargement because of it. After many years of carrying the extra burden, the overworked heart muscle may fail, with resultant symptoms of shortness of breath due to lung congestion and such evidences of fluid retention (edema) as swollen ankles. The arteries everywhere show involvement: atherosclerosis and degenerative changes appear much earlier than usual, a sort of premature aging of the vascular system.

Circulatory problems are all increased in individuals with hypertension: they show an increased incidence of strokes, heart attacks, and kidney difficulties.

Treatment. A variety of drugs and treatments have now changed the whole course of hypertension. Depending on the severity of the hypertension and the patient's response, various combinations of these drugs are employed. Among them are:

1. Rauwolfia derivatives—rauwolfia being the Indian root whose extract contains both tranquilizing and blood-pressure-lowering properties. The purified derivatives include reserpine (Serpasil®) and an agent called Singoserp®. These drugs may be sufficient for mild cases of hypertension; if not, other drugs can be added to the treatment program.

2. Diuretic drugs—a number of drugs known collectively as the chlorothiazide drugs—promote the excretion of salt and water by the kidneys. For reasons still unknown this also serves to lower blood pressure, sometimes quite effectively. These drugs may be given daily, produce an obvious increase in the amount of urine, and are basic drugs in the treatment of hypertension.

3. Apresoline—a drug which has no other equivalent—apparently acts on the brain centers that control blood pressure levels. It is often combined with the preceding drugs.

4. Ganglionic-blocking agents—drugs that block the transmission of nerve impulses to the small arteries which are narrowed in hypertension. As these small arteries dilate, the blood pressure levels drop.

BODY ODORS   Nature did not give the human body the pleasant odors she gave to the flowers—a situation partially rectified by perfume manufacturers. Although human sweat has practically no odor, it rather quickly develops one due to chemical changes produced by the ever-present bacteria on the skin. Such odorous changes are particularly likely to occur on the feet and between the toes, where a variety of organisms flourish. By removing the accumulation of materials on the skin surface (as well as many of the organisms), ordinary soap-and-water cleanliness makes a substantial contribution to decreasing odor.

Even more improvement can be achieved by using cleansing agents containing a medication known as hexachlorophene; this is a germ-killing agent which has a residual effect. Thus, when such substances are used day after day, the bacterial count of the skin diminishes markedly. (Hexachlorophene is the active ingredient often used by surgeons in scrubbing up prior to operations.) It is not generally necessary to use such agents over the entire surface, but they may be useful in special areas such as the feet, the groin, and the armpits. In the latter site the problem is further complicated by the presence of special glands whose secretion has a rather pungent odor. All individuals possess these glands, and in women, they have been shown to undergo changes throughout the menstrual cycle.

Most sprays, ointments, and liquids applied to the armpits contain aluminum salts. These decrease perspiration considerably and are sometimes combined with other agents which will decrease odor. Most of them work quite satisfactorily, although in individuals who perspire freely from the armpits, and especially in hot weather, more frequent applications may be necessary. A few individuals present special difficulties because of a condition of excessive perspiration, known as hyperhidrosis; the doctor may be able to suggest some special agents for controlling this.

Menstrual odors are by no means as common nor as marked as some hypersensitive women think. Appropriate powdering and frequent changes of napkins are of value. In some instances a tampon may be of further help. Masking scents (perfumes and powders with a pleasant odor of their own) can be helpful in concealing an objectionable odor.

▶ **Halitosis** Unpleasant odors on the breath are referred to as halitosis; these may be produced by diet, and are often only temporary after consumption of such items as liquor, onions and garlic, various spices, wines, etc. The degree to which halitosis is found objectionable varies with different groups; furthermore, if everyone partakes of the offending item, no one complains. Thus smokers generally have no objection to "tobacco breath," though non-smokers may complain. Poor mouth hygiene is sometimes a cause of halitosis and may require more frequent brushing of the teeth, perhaps combined with the use of dental floss or other cleansing techniques. Dentures should not be worn continuously and require cleaning from time to time.

Disordered digestion and certain conditions of the nose or respiratory passages may also make the breath odorous. The doctor will direct treatment to the underlying cause in these instances. Where the cause of an offensive odor cannot be tracked down or treated, a masking scent may be the only practical suggestion. Mints and similar items are, of course, widely used for such purposes.

BOILS AND CARBUNCLES   A boil is a local area of inflammation or abscess formation in the skin. A boil generally manifests itself initially as a hard, tender, reddish area. Later this softens; and if it comes to a "head," a variable amount of pus will be discharged. As compared to a pimple, a boil is somewhat larger and more deeply situated. A carbuncle is in turn larger still and involves more tissue destruction than a boil and, unlike the boil, a carbuncle has many heads through which pus may be discharged.

All three of these conditions may be regarded as basically interrelated, the common offending organism responsible for these suppurative infections of the skin being the staphylococcus organism. Since the staphylococcus is constantly found on the skin, it is not always possible to determine what has tipped the balance in favor of the invading germ. In some instances chafing or rubbing may be a factor, as when a boil develops under a tight collar or where the inner surfaces of the thighs rub against each other.

Boils sometimes develop in areas of the body where the circulation is less active, where sweating is excessive, as a complication of acne, or as a result of infection following the scratching of insect bites or other itching lesions of the skin. It is only infrequently that some systemic factor such as diabetes is found to be playing a role. Indeed, sometimes boils can be seen to come and go in crops in individuals who seem to be in excellent health.

A simple boil may not require much more attention than the application of hot wet compresses. These help to bring it to a head, and as a rule, once the pus has been discharged, progressive healing occurs without difficulty. If boils come and go frequently, more extensive treatment may be deemed desirable. This may include washing the skin with a soap containing an agent such as hexachlorophene, which destroys bacteria and has a residual effect also. In addition, antibiotics known to be effective against the staph group of organisms may be taken by mouth or in the form of ointments applied locally. Simple soap-and-water cleanliness seems to be all that is necessary in the handling of boils, and it is quite rare to see evidence of transmission of the bacteria in the usual boil from one member of a household to another. (See also ABSCESS.)

BRAIN DISORDERS IN CHILDREN

▶ **Brain Tumors** For purposes of description, the brain is divided roughly into two cerebral hemispheres and the posterior fossa (cerebellum, or brainstem). The dividing line between the hemispheres and brainstem is called the tentorium. In children, 60 to 70 per cent of brain tumors occur below the tentorium. Because of this difficult location, they cannot be completely removed. Sometimes they cannot even be reached.

The tumors are classified according to the area of the brain in which they occur and the particular cell type of tumor. The most frequently occurring brain tumors in childhood (75 per cent) are gliomas. About two-thirds of these are astrocytomas and medulloblastomas. The remainder are different forms of cell types. The location and cell pattern of the tumor determines whether the symptoms are major or minor. In infants under one or two years of age, a brain tumor will cause the head to get larger and produce signs of increasing intracranial pressure. This may become quite noticeable since the skull bones in the infant are soft and the suture lines allow growth and distention. As the head becomes large, there is compression of the brain due to the obstruction of the flow of cerebrospinal fluid. This fluid bathes the brain, its linings, and structures. When the pressure inside the brain has been markedly increased, the symptoms of headache, vomiting, weakness, lethargy, irritability, and poor appetite occur.

In children above three years of age, where the tumor is located in the cerebellum, signs of a disorder of balance occur. There may be a staggering gait (ataxia), tremors, swallowing and urinary difficulties, slurred speech, facial paralysis, cross-eyes, and other eye disorders. If the sixth nerve in the brain is involved, there may be loss of vision and nystagmus (horizontal or vertical oscillating eye movements), double vision, or complete blindness. Marked personality changes may occur. The signs may be temporary or progressive. Other disorders of equilibrium show in clumsiness and difficulty in handling toys. Playful and active children may become listless and lethargic. Other neurological signs depend upon the specific nerves involved. They are called *focal signs*. It is essential to hospitalize all children in whom such a diagnosis is suspected.

▶ **Organic Brain Damage** Behavior problems in children often reflect certain real and serious organic brain damage. Not all behavior disturbances are "psychological." A damaged or defective child has difficulty in the entire area of perceiving, learning, repeating, and reproducing desired behavior. These children are characteristically restless, hyperactive, easily excited, and easily distracted. They show unpredictable variations in their behavior, alternating from fairly normal to unpredictable, with outbursts of anger, destructiveness, and irritability. They often provoke fights, or tease and annoy others without cause. They are impulsive and act without thinking. They have difficulty in learning the concepts of reward, punishment, and competition. They have severe learning problems characterized by inability to pay attention for a prolonged period of time, difficulty with abstract thinking (particularly reading and arithmetic) and inability to form "concepts."

Only properly given psychological tests can determine whether these children are defective or damaged. There are special treatment methods for children who have difficulties in any of these learning areas. Retraining is the treatment of choice.

▶ **Hydrocephalus** Hydrocephalus is a condition characterized by an increase in the accumulation of cerebrospinal fluid in the brain. The cerebrospinal fluid represents a lake between the arteries and the brain and is the fluid which bathes the membranes of the brain. If there is some obstruction, or block, to the passage of this fluid, a dam is set up in which the fluid pressure builds up, causing a rapid increase in size of the head, with a separation of the bony sutures. The scalp veins become distended and the spaces between the bones (fontanels) become markedly enlarged. Growth and development are retarded. Increased pressure on the brain may also cause neurological symptoms.

Another form of hydrocephalus is called "communicating." This is the most common form; the block is in the intracranial subarachnoid space.

The imbalance occurs because absorption of cerebrospinal fluid does not equal its production; the head becomes quite spherical due to the increased cerebrospinal pressure. Treatment is therefore directed to getting rid of the excess cerebrospinal fluid. It is best to treat this condition as early as possible. Diagnosis is by X-ray and spinal tap.

Treatment is usually by means of some form of shunt or insertion of a polyethylene valve or tube which will permit the cerebrospinal fluid to drain into another area. Many cases of hydrocephalus remain minimal and require no surgical interference.

▶ **Mongolism (Down's Syndrome)** This is the name given to a type of mental retardation in which the child is born with certain typical characteristics: The eyes slant upward and outward, and the eye sockets are smaller than normal. The nose is small with an underdeveloped bridge, and the tongue usually protrudes. The fifth finger is short and in-curved, and the first and second toes are spaced widely apart. The skin may be dry with poor muscle tone and marked looseness of the joints. Mongoloid children are usually affectionate and pleasant but do not develop beyond the level of idiot or moron. They are very susceptible to infections and have a higher than average rate of leukemia.

The cause of mongolism is a specific chromosome abnormality. Sometimes the chromosomes number forty-seven instead of the normal forty-six, and an abnormally shaped chromosome may be found (Philadelphia chromosome). The condition is hereditary. Mongoloid children account for about 7 to 10 per cent of institutionalized mental defectives.

There is no treatment except home or institutionalized care, with recognition that these children are permanently retarded. The families are usually warned that they may possibly give birth to other children with this abnormality. (See also INTELLIGENCE—Mental Retardation.)

BRAIN, INFLAMMATION AND INFECTION

▶ **Encephalitis** Encephalitis means an inflammation of the brain. The symptoms consist of either gradual or sudden headache, fever, drowsiness, lethargy, and coma. In infants, convulsions may occur. Sometimes bizarre symptoms such as hyperactivity, nervousness, mental disorders, palsies, speech disorders, weakness, instability, and reflex changes are seen.

Encephalitis, like meningitis, may be caused by many different organisms. Some of them are: the virus of measles, infectious mononucleosis, insect-borne viruses, entero viruses, herpes, mumps, and smallpox virus. Other forms are: influenzal virus, lymphocytic choriomeningitis, St. Louis encephalitis, equine encephalitis, epidemic encephalitis, Von Economo's disease (encephalitis lethargica). There is no specific treatment for these diseases. However, patients should be in the hospital for supportive and symptomatic treatment.

Encephalitis may resemble poisonings with various metals such as lead, insecticides, etc., and drug intoxications, such as bromides, etc. In these cases, however, there is usually no fever.

▶ **Meningitis** Meningitis is an acute infectious disease of the meninges, or linings covering the brain.

Cause. Any number of different organisms, such as meningococcus, streptococcus, staphylococcus, pneumococcus, tubercle bacilli, and influenzal and a variety of other viruses.

Incubation period. Varies depending on infecting organism.

Symptoms. These vary slightly, depending upon the causative organisms. In general, however, in young children the most striking symptoms are: severe headache, fever, and great irritability and crankiness, particularly on being touched or bothered. There may be nausea, vomiting, and usually a stiff neck is a prominent sign. Convulsions and coma are often seen. Any child who has these complaints should be hospitalized immediately, and a spinal tap performed to confirm or rule out the diagnosis. A spinal tap is a procedure in which some of the spinal fluid is withdrawn by a syringe for study of the cell count, bacterial culture, and pressure.

The symptoms of meningitis frequently resemble those of polio, therefore a physician should always be called when any of these conditions is suspected. Various antibiotics are available to treat and usually cure meningitis. There is no specific immunization for meningitis. During epidemics, however, antibiotics may be used prophylactically to prevent cases.

BREASTS The breasts are made up of a large number of glands which, when stimulated, produce milk. They are supported in a framework of connective tissue and fat. The size and shape of the breasts are determined particularly by the supporting elements, and in the non-pregnant state the glandular elements may be relatively inconspicuous. A variety of factors will affect breast size. Hereditary factors which determine body build are sometimes obvious determinants of breast size also. Thus in some families many of the women run to large busts, in others to small busts, and this regardless of such features as height and even, to a lesser extent, of weight. In general, however, breast size will vary up and down parallel to body weight.

The glands of the breasts have a series of ducts or canals which converge toward the areola, the pigmented circular area surrounding the nipple. Here the ducts merge with one another and curve in so as to converge on the nipple. The actual openings of the milk ducts are scattered over the end of the nipple. Sometimes a nipple instead of protruding from the end of the breast may be virtually flush with the skin surface or even beneath it, a condition known as inverted nipple.

The glandular tissue of the breasts goes through cycles of growth and stimulation with every menstrual cycle. Just as the lining of the uterus is stimulated by the ovarian hormones, so too stimulation of the glandular elements of the breasts occurs. The degree to which this happens is more marked with some women and in some cycles than in others. However, it may be sufficient to result in obvious swelling of the breasts, and tenderness, which is most noticeable for a few days before menstruation. In pregnancy the breasts enlarge considerably because of specific and often intense stimulation of the glandular elements in preparation for nursing. Small amounts of secretion may collect on the nipple and dry there. This is known as colostrum, and need only be washed away with soap and warm water. (See also CHILDBIRTH—Delivery, Breasts After Delivery.)

▶ **Breasts, Tumors of** Various disorders of the glands and ducts may lead to tumors in the breasts. One such condition, considered to be due to unusual hormonal stimulation, is known as chronic cystic mastitis or fibrocystic disease. It is perhaps the most common cause of painful breasts in women, with the pain being most marked in the days prior to the menstrual period. The pain is usually felt in both breasts, the breasts are tender to palpation, and generally feel as though they were filled with shot. Usually all of these findings improve with the onset of menstruation; moreover, the condition can vary from one menstrual cycle to the next.

Sometimes one or several larger tumors may be found in the breasts. They may be marble-sized, generally are not tender, and are known as fibroadenomata. The more serious tumors of the breasts generally do not produce pain at all, and are often felt accidentally or incidentally, as for example while soaping in a shower. More serious tumors of the breasts are hard and sometimes produce a dimpling of the overlying skin.

It is often not possible to make a correct diagnosis of a lump in the breast without removing a portion of it for examination under the microscope. This procedure is called a biopsy. A woman who finds a lump in her breast should know first of all that even an expert may not be sure of its exact nature without such a biopsy, hence she is in no position to pass judgment on it herself. Secondly, she should be cautioned against unnecessary delay in establishing a diagnosis, and not allow precious time to pass in waiting for it to go away.

BRONCHITIS   The windpipe or trachea divides into a right and a left main stem bronchus in the upper part of the chest. These two major bronchi further subdivide into a system of pipelike channels which go to the five lobes into which the two lungs are divided (three on the right, two on the left). Within each lobe of the lung the bronchi undergo further division, and with each subdivision the size of the channel diminishes. This whole complex of branching tubes is referred to as the bronchial tubes and infection within them is termed bronchitis.

The many forms of bronchitis differ a great deal. Perhaps the chief thing they have in common is the symptom of cough, a prime indicator that something is going on in the trachea or bronchi. Thus certain viral inflammations of the respiratory tract, often termed tracheobronchitis, may produce relatively little phlegm but a good deal of irritative cough, so that people sometimes refer to "dry bronchitis" and the doctor to a non-productive cough. Various bacterial inflammations, however, will cause a great deal of phlegm production. The phlegm may be thick, yellowish or greenish white, and abundant amounts may be brought up with each cough. Rattling sounds may be produced by the flapping about of mucus with breathing and coughing, and the abundant phlegm or coughing is spoken of as a productive cough.

Since many viral inflammations may be succeeded by mixed infections with various bacteria, it is not uncommon to see a change from the dry hacking cough to a more productive one as a respiratory illness progresses. Indeed, occasionally a further stage is reached which is the extension of the bronchial infection down into the finer subdivisions of the lung—at which point we can speak of pneumonia or bronchopneumonia. Still another form of bronchitis can be produced by inhalation of irritant gases and fumes. The most common example of this is produced by cigarette smoking, which is by far the most frequent cause of chronic bronchitis.

▶ **Bronchitis, Chronic** It is often easier to clear up a pneumonia than to clear up a bronchitis. One reason for this is that pneumonia occurs in the lung substance proper and the antibiotic drugs which are administered can be brought to this region in large amounts. It is not possible to attain the same concentration of the antibiotic inside the larger bronchial tubes, so that inflammation here is resolved with greater difficulty.

In a few individuals wheezing due to narrowing and spasm of the bronchial tubes may occur in association with infection. This is spoken of as asthmatoid bronchitis, since it bears some resemblance to bronchial asthma. Indeed, somewhat similar drugs are used in the treatment of both conditions.

Treatment. Treatment will consist of cessation of smoking and the administration of antibiotics and other appropriate drugs. Sometimes special medicinal agents designed to liquefy the mucus may be administered. Maintaining a high humidity in room air, as for example by vaporizers, may be useful in all forms of bronchitis. It is clear that any form of bronchitis that hangs on, is associated with wheezing, or keeps recurring should be brought to the doctor's attention. (See also ASTHMA.)

BURNS   Burns are generally described in terms of their extent and the depth of the injury produced by heat. A burn of the back, for example, would be classified as an 18 per cent burn, one of the upper extremity as a 9 per cent burn. The depth of injury is classified in degrees: a *first degree burn* produces reddening of the skin; a *second degree burn* produces blistering; a *third degree burn* extends below the surface of the skin and produces injury to underlying tissues.

First and second degree burns, unless very extensive, can be treated in the doctor's office or in the home; third degree burns must be treated in a hospital setting. Immediate first aid may be helpful in cutting down the degree of injury due to a burn. Thus, if someone spills hot coffee over his hand, immediate immersion in cold running water might diminish the injury and would certainly help relieve the pain. Burns of the hands are usually quite painful, but pain can be relieved by immersing the hand in ice cold water. Such immersion for relief of pain can be maintained off-and-on for as long as seems necessary.

Blisters on the hands and the fingers are a fairly common second degree injury. When large, they are nuisances since they interfere with the use of the fingers. There is no reason why they should not be evacuated, and collapse of the blister actually promotes the rate of healing. In the doctor's office they will be aspirated by the use of a syringe and a small needle. If they are treated at home, it is best to start by painting the blister with a germ-killing solution. One end of the blister can then be pierced with a needle that has been flamed or dipped into alcohol for several minutes and then allowed to dry, and the fluid allowed to run out. It is best to prick the end of the blister which will be in the lowermost position when the hand is kept in the usual down position. First and second degree burn areas should be covered with vaseline and a dressing. Some of the common ointments available for first-aid use in the kitchen contain tannic acid, which should be applied only to very small areas and never to the face or genital regions.

CANCER ' New cells are constantly being formed in the body. Where replacement needs are high, as in the skin, the intestine, or the bone marrow (blood formation), the cells may be found multiplying at a correspondingly high rate. The new cells take their proper place and function. This kind of growth is orderly and necessary.

In cancer, the growth process goes astray. Here the new cells may not be organized properly, perform no useful function and, on the contrary, may destroy neighboring normal cells by the pressure they exert. A group of cancer cells may lie dormant for years or may for unknown reasons enlarge rapidly. At first the growth is local only. It may remain that way, and sometimes very large growths are encountered still in their site of origin. Some cancers, however, do not conform to normal boundary lines. Groups of cells may slip away and show up in a distant location, an event known as metastasis. Some cancers have been successfully treated even after metastasis has occurred. But generally once the growth has metastasized, the golden opportunity for cure is gone. Hence the emphasis on early detection, when the growth is still localized and cure can be achieved.

It should be remembered that the term "cancer" covers a whole spectrum of growths. Some are progressive, others very slow-growing. Some may pose relatively little threat—as, for example, the fairly common cancers of the skin and some of the cancers arising in the thyroid gland and the prostate gland. Acute leukemia in a child is a most serious illness, but chronic lymphatic leukemia in an elderly person is compatible with years of uneventful existence.

Although this variability may produce uncertainty in dealing with cancer, it also leads to hope. In general, the layman is more pessimistic about cancer than the doctor, who knows that many cancers can be cured and others can be lived with. Significant advances continue to be made; among them are the relatively recent discoveries that cancer of the lung can be largely avoided by abstaining from cigarette smoking, that early curable cancer of the uterus can be readily detected, and that even advanced cancer of the breast and of the prostate can show considerable response to hormonal drugs.

▶ **Hodgkin's Disease (Lymphogranulomatosis)** This is a malignant tumor whose cause is unknown. It affects the lymph nodes and lymphatic system. The spleen and lymph nodes enlarge and weakness, loss of weight and appetite usually occur. The nodes may enlarge in the neck or groin. Microscopic examination of the tissue of these enlarged nodes will give the diagnosis.

Treatment is usually radical surgery followed by X-ray. There are many new drugs which have proven useful in delaying what is ultimately a poor prognosis. However, there have been some long survivals.

▶ **Leukemia** This is a fatal disease suspected of being caused by a virus. It is characterized by uncontrolled production of white blood cells and of their immature forms. Leukemias are classified according to the predominant cell type which is involved, and also according to whether they are acute or chronic. Lymphocytes, monocytes, and myelocytes are most commonly involved. The disease is seen most frequently in the first five years of childhood, also in the eighth to ninth years.

The general symptoms are fever, weakness, weight loss, fatigue, pallor, bleeding, frequent and repeated infections, and easy bruising. The lymph nodes and the spleen may be enlarged. Bleeding from the mucous membranes (mouth) should make one suspicious of this condition. Normally, the white blood count is 8,000 to 10,000 cells/cu. mm. In leukemias there are blood counts of 200,000 cells per cubic mm. and more. Immature forms of white blood cells are often seen in the peripheral blood smears.

Modern treatment of leukemias with various chemicals has arrested some of the more acute cases. There are also some cases which remain chronic for many years. However, this disease does not have a very good long-term prognosis.

▶ **Neuroblastoma** Neuroblastoma is one of the most common malignant tumors in children. It is a tumor of the peripheral nerve cells derived from primitive sympathetic nerve tissue. Many arise from adrenal tissue or the chain of glands along the posterior portion of the chest. Their cell type varies, as does their degree of malignancy. The most frequent symptom is that of an abdominal tumor mass. If the tumor is very small, other symptoms such as fever, high white blood count, or a spread of this tumor to bone, liver, or eye, may occur. It is often found on both sides of the body, in contrast to another malignant tumor of childhood called Wilms' tumor. A sample of diseased tissue is examined under the microscope to determine the diagnosis.

Present treatment includes X-ray therapy and surgical excision followed by administration of various chemicals (chemotherapy) such as nitrogen mustard or antimetabolites.

▶ **Wilms' Tumor** This is a tumor of the kidney which arises from the embryonal cells. It is the most common kidney tumor in children, occurs during the first four years of life, and is usually limited to one side. It is one of the most common abdominal tumors of the early years.

The first sign is that of an enlarging abdomen. Other signs, such as blood in the urine, painful urination, anemia, fever, malnutrition, high blood pressure, constipation, etc., may arouse suspicion of this area. Wilms' tumor most frequently spreads to the lungs.

Surgical removal is followed by X-ray treatment and chemotherapy. There are many new drugs which have been used with some success in arresting this tumor. In general, however, the prognosis is poor.

CANCER, DETECTION OF

About half of all the cancer found in women is in relatively accessible locations where early detection is possible—in the breast where it can be detected by palpation or by special X-ray methods, and in the cervix where it can be detected by the "Pap" smear method.

In other organs cancer sometimes makes its presence known by departures from normal functioning. Thus cancer of the digestive tract may produce alterations in appetite, in capacity for food, or change in bowel habits such as constipation and diarrhea. Symptoms such as these, particularly in middle-aged and older individuals, may call for appropriate X-ray studies.

An annual physical examination—whether or not there are symptoms of any kind—is highly desirable. Many doctors feel that every woman should have a check of her breasts and of her reproductive organs twice a year, particularly past the age of thirty or thirty-five. Early localized cancer is in most instances readily cured, either with surgery or by X-ray. The American Cancer Society has issued a useful list in its program of education. Its early warning signals are the following:

1. Unusual bleeding or discharge.
2. A lump or thickening in the breast or elsewhere.
3. A sore that does not heal.

4. Change in bowel or bladder habits.
5. Persistent hoarseness or cough.
6. Persistent indigestion or difficulty in swallowing.
7. Change in a wart or mole.

▶ **"Pap" Smear** This is a cancer detection procedure developed by the Greek-American anatomist George Papanicolaou. The basic principle derives from the observation that in many locations in the body a growing tumor, just like adjacent normal tissue, will undergo some shedding of surface cells. When placed on a slide, stained, and examined under a microscope, it is possible to distinguish between normal and suspicious or obviously malignant cells. As a routine procedure, the "Pap" smear has been most successful when applied to the study of the uterus, particularly the cervix.

It seems both theoretically and practically possible to wipe out cancer of the cervix by routinely doing "Pap" smears on all women. It has been clearly shown that the "Pap" smear will pick up very early stages of cancer of the cervix, at a time when cure is relatively easy. In fact the "Pap" smear technique has demonstrated that this early non-invasive stage goes on for some years, throughout which time the "Pap" smear is consistently positive although nothing may be seen on naked-eye inspection.

The "Pap" smear procedure is very simple: a speculum is inserted into the vagina as is customarily done in routine pelvic examinations. The cervix, which protrudes into the upper part of the vagina, is thereby readily visualized. An ordinary cotton-tipped swab is inserted into the opening of the cervix, briefly rotated and removed. The swab is then streaked across an ordinary microscope slide. This can be stained at any convenient time thereafter.

By one system of classification the findings under the microscope are grouped into a series of grades ranging from 1 to 5. Class 1 is clearly normal, class 5 is clearly a malignant tumor; intermediate stages are suspicious and may require repeated follow-up or perhaps a biopsy of the cervix for further clarification. A negative "Pap" smear does not necessarily rule out disease, but when correctly done the "Pap" smear is a valuable cancer detection technique which should be far more widely employed.

CANKER SORE (APTHOUS STOMATITIS)   This mouth condition occurs both in children and adults. It is caused by the virus of *herpes simplex*. The lesions are characterized by groups of blisters which become ulcerated. They appear on the mucous membranes of the lips, cheeks, and tongue. Sometimes they extend into the throat area and involve the tonsils. The gums frequently start to swell and bleed.   They may cause fever and swollen glands. Eating becomes painful and difficult. Prophylaxis and proper mouth hygiene are important in preventing this condition. Since it is contagious, the eating utensils should be kept separate and boiled.

Treatment. Treatment is with bland diet, mild antiseptic mouth washes and antibiotics by injection and by mouth. Penicillin and aureomycin have been used with success. The ulcers may also be treated locally with applications of silver nitrate, a caustic agent which helps to heal them. The condition usually clears within five to seven days.

CATHETERIZATION   Catheterization is the passing of a plastic or rubber tube into a channel or hollow organ of the body. The most common kind of catheterization is performed on the urinary bladder. It is done most often because of inability to urinate, which may be encountered after a general anesthetic or after childbirth. In men difficulty in urinating is most often due to enlargement of the prostate.

Catheterization used to be done almost routinely during deliveries, and not infrequently afterwards, if the need arose. However, it is best to try other alternatives such as the following: hot compresses or ice-cold compresses to the pubic region; running a water tap; bypassing the bedpan in favor of the commode or toilet. In some cases it is necessary to keep a catheter in the bladder for some time. It may be referred to as an "inlying catheter." One form of this is the Foley catheter, which has a small balloon. After this is inflated it will keep the catheter securely situated within the bladder.

▶ **Cardiac Catheterization** Cardiac catheterization is a procedure which has been developed over recent years for evaluating disorders of the heart. It is used particularly to evaluate the departures from normal in congenital heart disease, or in estimating the degree of damage in a rheumatic heart. In cardiac catheterization a very long catheter is passed up the vein into a heart chamber, where pressure measurements can be taken and samples withdrawn for analysis of oxygen content. Cardiac catheterization is an invaluable diagnostic aid that is performed almost routinely before cardiac surgery.

CELIAC SYNDROME   Celiac syndrome combines a number of specific symptoms which occur in children who are unable to digest starches or fats, or both. In cases of fat intolerance, there will be a defect in the absorption of fatty acids from the intestines. There may be a single defect, the absorption of starch, or, there may be a combination of both. A more severe form of the latter is called cystic fibrosis of the pancreas.

Celiac disease is a chronic nutritional disturbance occurring generally from the age of ten months to five years. Children affected with this condition fail to grow and thrive. They develop enlarged protuberant abdomens with weak, wasted muscles, particularly in the buttocks and extremities. They show evidence of vitamin deficiencies and pass large, bulky, foul-smelling stools. The stools will float if they are placed in water because of their large fat and starch content. These children are extremely cranky and irritable. Even though they may be receiving adequate food and nutrition, they are really malnourished, suffering from a serious defect in the absorption of foods. Normal stool contains a fat content of approximately 20 per cent or even less. Celiac stools contain anywhere from 30 to 60 per cent fat. The body is unable to absorb and utilize this fat; therefore, it has to be excreted.

As a result of the absorption deficiency, rickets, thinning of the bones (osteoporosis), hemorrhagic disease due to vitamin K deficiency, and secondary anemias develop.

Celiac disease has been shown to be a deficiency in absorption of gliadin, which is the active ingredient found in the protein fraction of wheat (gluten). Feeding even small amounts of gluten to children with celiac disease will induce severe diarrhea crises. A slice of bread or a cracker will cause abdominal pain, vomiting, and shock within hours. Most investigators feel that starch plays a more significant role than fat in the development of celiac syndrome.

Treatment. Celiac disease is treated with the Dorothy Anderson diet which starts with protein milk and banana powder, then graduates to scraped beef and tomato juice, ripe bananas, pot cheese, gelatin, squash, peas, celery, spinach. As improvement occurs, other meats, eggs, baked apples, and vegetables are added to the diet. Toast, bread, cereals, potatoes, whole milk, and butter are the very last to be added.

True cures of this condition are rare, and one generally speaks of remission rather than cure.

CERVIX   The cervix is the lowest, narrowed portion of the uterus, and projects into the upper part of the birth canal (vagina). The normal cervix has a pink-white, solid appearance which is quite uniform. At its center is a small opening —the "os" or mouth—which leads into a narrow canal running the length of the cervix and entering the uterine cavity. A sampling of the tissue within the os, generally taken by a swab and placed on a microscope slide, is the basis of the "Pap" smear, an important diagnostic procedure for cancer. (See CANCER—Pap Smear.)

Many contraceptive devices and techniques act as barriers, preventing sperm from entering the os. In a non-pregnant woman it is a small circular opening; after one or more deliveries, however, it is larger and may appear as a slightly irregular slit running transversely. Women who use a diaphragm become familiar with the firm consistency of the cervix. (See BIRTH CONTROL.)

One of the remarkable changes that occurs in delivery is the virtual disappearance of the cervix as an identifiable structure. When fully dilated at the time of delivery, the opening of the cervix permits the baby's head to descend into the vagina. That this thin-walled and distended segment can return within a matter of weeks to a size and shape somewhat resembling that before pregnancy is truly remarkable. (See CHILDBIRTH AND PREGNANCY—Labor.)

Infection within the cervix known as endocervicitis may lead to a mucous discharge. There may (sometimes in association with endocervicitis, but also independently) be a change in the appearance of the cervical tissue adjacent to the os. Instead of a dull opaque white, the os may appear thinner and redder; this is known as erosion. The doctor will often treat endocervicitis and erosion by a procedure known as cauterization, which promotes the return of the tissue to normal.

CHICKEN POX (VARICELLA)   Contagious.

Cause. Virus.

Incubation period. 2 to 3 weeks.

Symptoms. Slight illness, including loss of appetite, feelings of malaise, and mild fever, may be present before the rash breaks out. The rash starts with small, red, flat patches which become raised and then blistered. The blisters fill with cloudy fluid. There are all stages of eruption present at the same time. It appears first on the body, then spreads to the face and head (including mucous membranes of the mouth, vulva, etc.). Very few pox appear on the legs and arms. After the fluid-filled blisters dry, they crust and become scabs. If the child scratches them, they may become infected. The rash, which causes severe itching, continues to break out for three to five days, and is often seen inside the mouth and in the hair.

The lymph glands in the body also become enlarged. Ear infections, pneumonia, and other complications have been known to follow this disease. There is no known prevention. However, one attack usually gives permanent immunity.

Treatment. Local starch baths, or starch applications, and soothing lotions and creams to suppress itching are helpful. Children should be prevented from picking the scabs off before they are completely dry, as ugly, pitted scars may result if they are prematurely loosened. It is advisable not to give the child a complete tub bath until all the scabs have fallen off. Premature soaking will only loosen them and cause scars. A physician should always be called to determine whether the case is chicken pox or smallpox, which it resembles. However, smallpox is rarely seen in this country due to mass vaccination programs.

CHILDBIRTH AND PREGNANCY

▶ **Pregnancy Tests** Most of the pregnancy tests used are based upon the observation that large amounts of hormones are produced when pregnancy occurs. These hormones are secreted by the developing embryo; they are passed on into the blood of the mother and some are excreted through the kidney and urine. Hence pregnancy tests can be done on either blood or urine specimens.

The particular hormones tested for are known as the gonadotropins, hormones which stimulate the sex glands—the ovaries or the testes. In the case of the commonly performed Friedman's test (Friedman-Lapham test, or rabbit test) the course of events is as follows: It is known that the isolated female rabbit has in her ovaries ripe follicles ready to shed their eggs. Injection of a small amount of an ovary-stimulating hormone, such as may be found in the urine or blood of a pregnant woman, will produce rupture of these follicles with release of their eggs—ovulation. The test is simple to perform. An extract of an overnight urine specimen or the serum of a blood specimen from the pregnant woman is injected into the rabbit's ear vein. Twenty-four hours later an abdominal incision is made and the rabbit's ovaries inspected. If ovulation has occurred, the alteration in the appearance of the ovary is easily seen by naked-eye inspection. This would be a positive pregnancy test.

There are other forms of pregnancy testing which include: (1) the original A-Z (Aschheim-Zondek) test, based upon observation of stimulation by the pregnant woman's hormones of the immature testes or ovaries of a rat; (2) the frog or toad test, based upon the fact that these same hormones of pregnancy will produce extrusion of sperm in a frog or a toad. The frog test may be read within a few hours. Recently new pregnancy tests have been devised which do away with experimental animals altogether. They are based upon delicate testing of the immunization type.

None of these tests is 100 per cent accurate very early in pregnancy. But this level of accuracy is almost reached two weeks or more after the menstrual period is missed. Hence a positive test means more than a negative test, and a negative test does not always rule out the possibility of early pregnancy. If other signs indicate a possible pregnancy and a first test is reported negative, another test should be run.

TABLE OF THE DURATION OF PREGNANCY

Month	Day numbers	→
January	1 2 3 4 5 6 7 8 9 10 11 12 13 14 15 16 17 18 19 20 21 22 23 24 25 26 27 28 29 30 31	
October ...	8 9 10 11 12 13 14 15 16 17 18 19 20 21 22 23 24 25 26 27 28 29 30 31 1 2 3 4 5 6 7	November
February	1 2 3 4 5 6 7 8 9 10 11 12 13 14 15 16 17 18 19 20 21 22 23 24 25 26 27 28	
November ...	8 9 10 11 12 13 14 15 16 17 18 19 20 21 22 23 24 25 26 27 28 29 30 1 2 3 4 5	December
March	1 2 3 4 5 6 7 8 9 10 11 12 13 14 15 16 17 18 19 20 21 22 23 24 25 26 27 28 29 30 31	
December ..	6 7 8 9 10 11 12 13 14 15 16 17 18 19 20 21 22 23 24 25 26 27 28 29 30 31 1 2 3 4 5	January
April	1 2 3 4 5 6 7 8 9 10 11 12 13 14 15 16 17 18 19 20 21 22 23 24 25 26 27 28 29 30	
January	6 7 8 9 10 11 12 13 14 15 16 17 18 19 20 21 22 23 24 25 26 27 28 29 30 31 1 2 3 4	February
May	1 2 3 4 5 6 7 8 9 10 11 12 13 14 15 16 17 18 19 20 21 22 23 24 25 26 27 28 29 30 31	
February	5 6 7 8 9 10 11 12 13 14 15 16 17 18 19 20 21 22 23 24 25 26 27 28 1 2 3 4 5 6 7	March
June	1 2 3 4 5 6 7 8 9 10 11 12 13 14 15 16 17 18 19 20 21 22 23 24 25 26 27 28 29 30	
March	8 9 10 11 12 13 14 15 16 17 18 19 20 21 22 23 24 25 26 27 28 29 30 31 1 2 3 4 5 6	April
July	1 2 3 4 5 6 7 8 9 10 11 12 13 14 15 16 17 18 19 20 21 22 23 24 25 26 27 28 29 30 31	
April	7 8 9 10 11 12 13 14 15 16 17 18 19 20 21 22 23 24 25 26 27 28 29 30 1 2 3 4 5 6 7	May
August	1 2 3 4 5 6 7 8 9 10 11 12 13 14 15 16 17 18 19 20 21 22 23 24 25 26 27 28 29 30 31	
May	8 9 10 11 12 13 14 15 16 17 18 19 20 21 22 23 24 25 26 27 28 29 30 31 1 2 3 4 5 6 7	June
September	1 2 3 4 5 6 7 8 9 10 11 12 13 14 15 16 17 18 19 20 21 22 23 24 25 26 27 28 29 30	
June	8 9 10 11 12 13 14 15 16 17 18 19 20 21 22 23 24 25 26 27 28 29 30 1 2 3 4 5 6 7	July
October	1 2 3 4 5 6 7 8 9 10 11 12 13 14 15 16 17 18 19 20 21 22 23 24 25 26 27 28 29 30 31	
July	8 9 10 11 12 13 14 15 16 17 18 19 20 21 22 23 24 25 26 27 28 29 30 31 1 2 3 4 5 6 7	August
November	1 2 3 4 5 6 7 8 9 10 11 12 13 14 15 16 17 18 19 20 21 22 23 24 25 26 27 28 29 30	
August	8 9 10 11 12 13 14 15 16 17 18 19 20 21 22 23 24 25 26 27 28 29 30 31 1 2 3 4 5 6	September
December	1 2 3 4 5 6 7 8 9 10 11 12 13 14 15 16 17 18 19 20 21 22 23 24 25 26 27 28 29 30 31	
September ..	7 8 9 10 11 12 13 14 15 16 17 18 19 20 21 22 23 24 25 26 27 28 29 30 1 2 3 4 5 6 7	October

The numbers in the first line represent the first day of the last menstrual period. The second line gives the estimated date of parturition.

75

▶ **Fetal Development** This term refers to the growth of the unborn baby. Its development in the uterus during the 280 days following the missed menstrual period is the greatest and most complex growth process in nature. It transforms the tiny fertilized ovum, invisible to the naked eye, into the six-to-eight pound human infant whose lusty birth cry marks the appearance of a new human being. Development proceeds somewhat as follows, with times representing averages from the first day of the last menstrual period:

14 days—sperm penetrates the egg, fertilization

14-17 days—fertilized egg proceeds down the tube

24 days—fertilized egg, now a little ball of cells, burrows into the lining of uterus

30 days—embryo well embedded in uterine lining. Multiple little processes have sprouted like roots for taking up nourishment.

6 weeks—head, spinal canal, and vertebrae forming. Rudiments of eyes, ears, and nose have appeared.

8 weeks—one inch long. Head is proportionately large, rudimentary extremities. Eyes, face, and features forming.

12 weeks—3 inches long. Arms, legs, hands, and feet formed. Distinct fingers and toes with soft nails. External sex organs begin to show differences between male and female.

16 weeks—4-6 inches long; 2-4 ounces in weight. Fine downy hair (lanugo) covers skin. Obvious external sex organs.

20 weeks—12 inches long; ¾ of a pound in weight. Fetal movements begin, heart sounds may be heard by doctor.

24 weeks—1½ pounds in weight. Skin is wrinkled, eyebrows and lashes are formed. If child is born it cannot survive.

28 weeks—2½ pounds in weight. Eyes open. Well-developed head hair.

32 weeks (end of seventh month)—16 inches long; 3½ pounds in weight. The child looks like a "little old man," with not much fat in the skin.

36 weeks—18 inches long; 5 pounds in weight. Face is less wrinkled, because of fat deposits.

40 weeks (full term infant)—19-20 inches long; 6½-8 pounds in weight. Scalp hair is dark, the skin smooth

and covered with white secretion. There are well-developed nails and head hair. Eyes are slate-colored, but the final color cannot be predicted.

▶ **Prenatal Care** A routine form of professional care for a pregnant woman, generally given by a doctor or nurse, is called prenatal care. The objectives of prenatal care are to keep the mother as healthy as possible throughout the pregnancy, avoiding or minimizing the various disorders that may be associated with the pregnant state and insuring that the unborn baby is well nourished and developed. The routines involved may vary somewhat, as will the time and frequency of the visits.

Basic elements of prenatal care will include keeping track of weight, blood pressure and urine to avoid toxemia of pregnancy. Attention will be paid to diet since pregnancy calls for special measures such as increased calcium and iron as well as maintenance of a well-balanced high vitamin diet. Influenza and polio are somewhat more hazardous to women who are pregnant, and appropriate immunizations may be called for. The dangers of German measles, especially to the fetus, are well known. Swelling of the legs, development of varicose veins, obesity and vaginal infections may occur. (See VAGINITIS.) Heartburn, excess salivation, constipation, nausea and vomiting are some of the digestive problems frequently encountered. The doctor is able to treat or alleviate most of these.

▶ **"Morning Sickness"** A significant number of pregnant women experience nausea of varying degrees during the first third of their pregnancies. There is no doubt that some physical change in the digestive tract underlies this complaint. Thus women have been known to complain of nausea before they missed their menstrual period—i.e., before they had reason to believe they might be pregnant. Worries and anxieties about the pregnancy may increase complaints regarding nausea, much as tension may increase a headache or stomach cramps. In addition, anything that can produce or contribute to nausea in the non-pregnant state will do the same to a pregnant woman—whether it be an unpleasant sight or thought, greasy food, or unpleasant odors. The complaint is most marked on arising and shortly thereafter. Both physical and psychological factors may be involved in "morning sickness."

Treatment. Various procedures may be helpful:

1. Before retiring for the night, place two or three dry crackers at the bedside; these should be eaten on awakening in the morning without getting up. After a wait of twenty minutes or so, one can arise.

2. Overloading the stomach, particularly in the morning, should be avoided. Breakfast should be small and should be followed a few hours later by a mid-morning snack.

3. Avoid fats and fried or greasy foods.

4. All else being equal, a meal consisting largely of solids will sit more easily than one containing much fluid—it may be preferable to save the fluid intake for later in the day.

5. Various mild sedatives and tranquilizers will help allay nausea, but none should be taken without first checking with the doctor.

▶ **Toxemia of Pregnancy** This term refers to an abnormality found in the last two to three months of pregnancy and occasionally in the period immediately following the delivery. Its causes are unknown, but the condition is specific to pregnancy and is more common during first pregnancies, or if twins are present. It is sometimes impossible to distinguish mild degrees of this disorder from many of the normal events in pregnancy. As the doctor sees it, there is a rise in blood pressure, an unusual amount of edema (puffiness), and albumin in the urine.

The pregnant woman may feel entirely well but should be aware of the possibilities of toxemia if she undergoes rapid weight gain (on the order of two to three pounds per week), if the fingers swell up so that rings become tight, or if the face becomes puffy. Headaches or blurring of vision usually indicate that toxemia is well established. Any pregnant woman experiencing any of these symptoms should communicate with her doctor at once and not let matters slide until the next regular appointment. Toxemia is rare where there has been good prenatal care; when caught early, it is generally easily reversed.

Treatment. The measures that the doctor prescribes will include rest, restriction of salt in the diet, and perhaps also the taking of such drugs as the diuretics, which promote the excretion of fluid, or drugs designed to lower the blood pressure. If the blood pressure is unusually high, or if other findings warrant it, the doctor may well advise a few days' stay in the hospital for observation. Mild degrees of toxemia are by no means rare—especially toward the very end of pregnancy. That the condition is somehow related to secretions coming from the uterus, perhaps the placenta, is indicated by the usually prompt disappearance of the puffiness and the drop in blood pressure that occurs upon delivery.

► **Weight Gain in Pregnancy** It is the doctor's hope in most instances that the weight gain in pregnancy should not exceed twenty pounds. The exception would be a painfully thin woman for whom some filling-out would be desirable. For her, pregnancy may be a good opportunity to put on some desired weight. The twenty-pound figure for normal pregnancy gain is based on adding together the following: the baby, seven pounds; enlargement of the uterus, three pounds; placenta and uterine fluid, two pounds; increase in breast weight, up to two pounds. Adding approximately six pounds of retained fat and fluid to this total of fourteen pounds can be regarded as reasonable. During the first three months of pregnancy some women exhibit no weight gain because of nausea; others gain as much as four to five pounds. During the last six months of pregnancy the weight gain should not be at a rate faster than two-thirds to three-fourths of a pound per week. The rate at which this weight is gained fluctuates from week to week and cannot be exact. However, rapid weight gains such as one to two pounds per week—especially when accompanied by obvious puffiness of the face and around the eyes and by headaches—should be reported to the doctor.

Many women experience an inordinate stimulation of appetite during pregnancy. If intake is not restrained, very large weight gains are possible. A woman who throws caution to the winds can gain thirty to forty pounds and, of course, will find that putting it on is much easier than taking it off. It is wise to avoid extra weight gains in pregnancy beyond an upper limit of approximately twenty-four pounds.

► **The Pelvis and Childbirth** The bones that make up the pelvis are put together in such a manner as to form an oval basin-like enclosure. The largest of the bones, the innominate, extends from the sacrum in the midline of the back and forms a curve which runs up to the front and, again in the midline, meets the pubic bones. The junction of the two pubic bones in the midline in front is called the pubic symphysis. It is only some two inches in height and can be easily felt just above the genital region.

Late in pregnancy the pubic symphysis actually becomes looser and more mobile in preparation for the baby's birth. When looked at from below, the opening through the pelvis is much narrower; it is called the pelvic outlet. The size of the pelvic outlet is of major importance in obstetrics. If it is small, and if the baby's head is proportionately large, Caesarean section may be necessary.

Although it is impossible to measure the pelvic outlet precisely, the doctor can take a series of measurements of the pelvis at different points and draw quite accurate conclusions as to the size of the outlet. In a few cases (as when the pelvis has been deformed because of poliomyelitis with paralysis early in life) it may be obvious that normal delivery cannot be expected.

Sometimes the measurements taken by the doctor may be borderline, so that he cannot be sure whether a normal-sized baby can be delivered from below. The doctor may therefore decide to observe the course of labor before coming to a decision as to whether or not Caesarean section is necessary. This is known as "trial of labor." In the overwhelming percentage of cases, of course, such mechanisms as the loosening-up of the pubic symphysis, the relaxation of other ligaments binding the pelvis, and the molding of the baby's head will all be factors that will abet a normal delivery. Nature is often further aided when the doctor performs the procedure known as episiotomy.

▶ **Labor** The baby is brought into the world by painful contractions of the uterus. These pains are labor pains. Exactly what initiates them, after nine months of relative quiet, is unknown. In some women painful uterine contractions may occur for a period of some hours about a week or two before true labor begins. Such pains may even result in a woman's being brought to the hospital before the pains, instead of increasing, decrease and then disappear. This is sometimes referred to as "false labor."

In contrast, true labor pains are characterized by regular rhythmicity, increasing intensity, and a progressive shortening of the interval between contractions. It is sometimes wise to time the intervals between the pains to determine precisely whether the intervals are diminishing. As soon as it is clear that true labor pains have commenced, the doctor should be contacted. He is the one to determine the time at which hospitalization seems desirable. His decision in this respect will be influenced by the knowledge of whether or not this is a first baby, whether there is a history of rapid deliveries in the past, and whether a woman may not feel more secure in a hospital setting. The total duration of labor is generally somewhere between twelve and eighteen hours, but it can be either longer or shorter by another six hours. It is generally shorter in women who have had one or more previous children (multiparas, from *multi,* many; *para,* birth).

It is customary to divide labor into stages. In the *first stage* there is a gradual dilatation and softening-up of the cervix, the lowermost portion of the uterus which protrudes into the vagina. (See CERVIX.) The extent of this dilatation can be judged by rectal examination. When the opening of the cervix has reached approximately 2½ inches, the woman is said to be "fully dilated." Approximately 90 per cent of the total duration of the labor is involved in reaching this point. During the second stage of labor, the baby passes through the uterus and the vagina on his way into the outside world. The second stage may take one to two hours in a woman having her first baby, generally considerably less in others.

The *second stage* may tax the skill of the doctor and require good patient cooperation. Depending on how things are going, the doctor may ask the mother to bear down, which aids in the delivery process, or to avoid bearing down, perhaps to avoid a precipitate delivery with possible tissue damage. In the case of a breech delivery, the doctor may have to work rapidly. During the second stage the powerful uterine contractions may push the baby's head periodically up to the vaginal entrance, an event known as "crowning." At about this point the doctor may elect to do an episiotomy to widen the opening.

An episiotomy makes the delivery of the baby easier for both mother and infant. In hospital practice it is almost routine to do an episiotomy, especially for women having their first delivery. Another indication for doing an episiotomy would be evidence of undue stretching as the baby's head comes down, suggesting the possibility that a tear may occur. Instead of running the risk of such a tear, which may be irregular, deep, or lead to complications, an episiotomy will be done to control the threatening situation. Other advantages of episiotomy are: (1) It substitutes a surgical incision which is easily repaired for lacerations which may be difficult to repair. (2) It is easier on the baby's head and avoids some of the risk of damage to it. (3) It shortens labor.

The *third stage* of labor consists of delivery of the afterbirth or placenta. This generally takes about fifteen minutes and completes the act of labor.

CHILDBIRTH—DELIVERY

▶ **Natural Childbirth** Natural childbirth is a term generally used to describe a program of care and instruction during pregnancy which emphasizes physical and psychological preparation for the delivery. Its exponents have emphasized that feelings of fear and isolation, coupled with the complete ignorance about labor which used to be true of most women, lead to anxiety and muscular tension; these in turn increase the pain, may perhaps prolong the labor, and therefore increase the woman's difficulties. Natural childbirth has also emphasized the importance of a positive and supportive relationship between the woman in labor and those about her. Since isolation may increase the pain and anxiety, natural childbirth requires support for the woman in the labor room, which may include visiting by the husband.

Some hospitals sponsor classes of instruction based upon natural childbirth. There are lectures and demonstrations which discuss the anatomy of pregnancy and the mechanism of delivery. Instruction is also given in the various methods of breathing which will be of importance during labor. Systematic exercises and methods for producing relaxation, both of value during delivery, are part of the instruction. In some hospital settings the area of the unknown is further reduced by a tour through the obstetric wards, inspection of the labor rooms, and introduction to the nursing personnel who may be present at the time of delivery. There is generally one lecture for the expectant fathers.

Various books dealing with the subject of natural childbirth and descriptions of the exercises used are readily available. There can be no doubt that natural childbirth and programs derived from it have diminished previous fears based on ignorance and, therefore, diminish the impact of labor pains. Proponents of natural childbirth never claim that it can make labor a painless process, but rather that a woman who is not tense and who knows what is happening will experience considerably less discomfort. Thus natural childbirth does not mean that pain-killing drugs or anesthetics are unnecessary.

▶ **Caesarean Birth** A Caesarean birth is a delivery made through an incision into the abdomen and uterus. The most frequent reason for this kind of delivery is a contracted pelvis —a pelvis whose dimensions are too small to permit a normal (natural) delivery. Sometimes the operation is decided upon after a trial of labor indicates that vaginal delivery will be very difficult or impossible. However, if it has become clear that a Caesarean section will be necessary, the mother may be admitted to a hospital late in the ninth month of pregnancy and delivered by Caesarean procedure before labor pains have commenced. Such a planned Caesarean birth is known as an elective Caesarean section. It is often done on women who have had a previous Caesarean, the thought being that the scar into the uterus from the previous operation represents a weak spot and, therefore, a potentially troublesome one if labor is permitted.

"Once a Caesarean always a Caesarean" is still a pretty general rule. Accordingly, some women have had three, four, or even more babies by the Caesarean route. A Caesarean section is sometimes done after a too-early separation of the placenta (the afterbirth), since otherwise the baby's life is endangered. Still another reason might be a first pregnancy late in a woman's life: doing a Caesarean delivery may mean less of a risk to the baby, and in a sense will insure that the mother will have at least one successful pregnancy.

▶ **Breech Delivery** In about 3 per cent of all births, the legs or buttocks rather than the head present first. Such presentations are referred to as breeches. The reason for the breech presentation is unknown. Occasionally attempts may be made before the delivery to shift the baby's position within the womb into the head-down position. Once labor has begun, such a maneuver may not be possible. Unfortunately, even if it is successful at first, it may be found that the baby may again return to the breech position some time before the delivery.

83

A breech presentation makes the delivery somewhat more difficult from the doctor's point of view. So far as the mother is concerned no difference in the labor will be noted. Various technical maneuvers are available to the obstetrician in expediting the second stage of labor when a breech presentation occurs. In the delivery of twins or other multiple births, one or more of the babies may come out in the breech position. The problem here is eased somewhat, however, by the fact that the infants are generally smaller and hence more easily maneuvered.

▶ **The Umbilical Cord (Navel)** The umbilical cord is the cord through which nourishment is supplied to the fetus. The cord, containing a vein and two umbilical arteries, is attached to the mother's placenta and to the infant at the middle of the abdomen.

At birth, the cord is cut a few inches from the abdomen and clamped so that it does not bleed. It is permitted to dry, whereupon it falls off, leaving the depression known as the navel or "belly button." Sometimes the cord oozes pus or may separate and bleed a little. Pressure for five or ten minutes will stop the bleeding. The drainage from a healing cord can be cleansed with alcohol. Antibiotic ointments may also be required.

It is advisable not to bathe the infant in a tub until the cord has dried and fallen off, since it may become infected with dirty bath water. Sometimes there is incomplete closure of the inner portion of the cord, and a protrusion results. This is called an *umbilical hernia*. It usually enlarges when the infant strains at stool or cries. If it becomes very large, it runs the danger of becoming an *incarcerated umbilical hernia*. If this occurs, an emergency operation is required. Sometimes the doctor will advise taping the umbilical hernia with adhesive tape to prevent it from enlarging.

▶ **Premature Infants** An infant who weighs five and a half pounds or less is termed premature. This definition applies whether the child is born at the full nine months or earlier. Children who are born before term usually weigh less than normal and therefore, automatically, are called premature ("preemies"). These babies are generally a bit weaker than normal. They may cry in a more feeble manner; the skin is loose and wrinkled and their temperature is unstable and generally lower than normal. They may lose more weight in the beginning than heavier babies, and their general gain is not as rapid. They require extra warmth in an incubator and special precautions to prevent infection. Many premature infants require feeding from tubes (gavage feeding) or feeding from a dropper. Their sucking and swallowing reflexes and muscles are not well developed.

Premature babies have many other immature features. However, they generally catch up with full-term babies and their subsequent development is not necessarily damaged by the fact of their prematurity. Because of their anatomic and physiological immaturity, premature babies are particularly susceptible to many illnesses, including circulatory, respiratory, gastrointestinal, urinary, and other difficulties. Prematurity is the leading cause of infant deaths. The prevention of prematurity depends on excellent professional obstetrical care and on early diagnosis and treatment of conditions in the mother which may dispose to prematurity.

Premature infants are fed nothing by mouth during the first twenty-four to forty-eight hours. Then boiled sugar water (5 per cent solution) is given. Formulas for prematures should be high in protein, low in fat, and high in calcium. One-half powdered skim milk and one-half fresh skimmed or evaporated milk is generally used. In the second week, vitamins are added to the formula (vitamins A, B, and C). Most of these babies eat more often than every four hours in the beginning months. They may have more frequent bowel movements. This has sometimes been mistaken for "diarrhea" and caused alarm. It is not diarrhea, but is merely due to the infant's limited capacity. The frequency of movements lessens in time as the infant's capacity to hold more ounces of food grows.

▶ **Twins and Multiple Births** Twins occur approximately once in ninety births, triplets once in 9,300 pregnancies, quadruplets once in 490,000 pregnancies, and quintuplets approximately once in 8 million deliveries. The peak incidence for twins occurs in women between 35 and 40, is more common in women with previous pregnancies, more common in Negroes than in Caucasians, and is least common among the Japanese.

Most often twins come about because two eggs are released simultaneously rather than the usual one. The resulting offspring have no more resemblance to one another than is usual between brothers and sisters. They are referred to as fraternal (non-identical) twins. Occasionally a single fertilized egg can divide into two identical halves, each of which is capable of complete development. There then results a pair of what are called identical twins. Identical twins are always of the same genetic constitution and therefore have the same sex, look alike to the point of being difficult to tell apart, and possess the same temperament, intellect, etc.

In the case of triplets, quadruplets, and multiple births generally, any combination of fraternal or identical babies may be found in the offspring. Thus triplets may be identical, consist of two identical and one fraternal twin, or be derived from three separate eggs and be entirely fraternal. Since the babies are generally smaller in multiple births, the actual delivery may be physically easier. However, breech presentations and prematurity are often complicating factors.

▶ **Breasts After Delivery** The production of milk is the result of stimulation of the breasts by a pituitary hormone. This milk-producing principle is inhibited throughout pregnancy by the sex-hormone production of the placenta, the afterbirth, an interesting example of nature's wisdom. Thus during the latter part of pregnancy and for the first couple of days after the delivery, only a clear fluid known as colostrum may exude from the nipples. Milk production begins often in a dramatic way, about three days after the delivery. The breasts may suddenly become full, hard, and tender, an event known as engorgement. The network of veins may visibly develop in the skin of the breasts, becoming much more prominent.

If the decision is made to nurse the infant, the pain and fullness of the breast will promptly be helped by the breast feeding. This emptying of the breast is also a strong stimulus to further milk production. If the mother decides not to nurse, she may have some discomfort for several days while the breasts learn to adjust to this situation. Several steps may be of value during this time: (1) The pain of engorgement will be relieved by aspirin, codeine, or similar drugs. (2) Ice bags may be applied to the breasts, an hour on and an hour off. (3) A well-fitting snug bra giving uplift and support will be useful. (See also INFANT FEEDING.)

▶ **Care of Nipples** The nipples need no special care during pregnancy. However, if a nipple is flat or inverted, and especially if nursing is planned, the doctor or nurse may show procedures for bringing the nipple out and making it more prominent. One technique consists of cupping the hand around the areola—the pigmented circular area around the nipple—and gently pressing down the tissue around the nipple so as to make it more prominent. With the fingers of the other hand, the nipple can be gently pulled on and stripped. The procedure can be repeated for a minute or two; in conjunction with the enlargement that occurs during pregnancy anyway, a flat nipple can thus be "brought out" reasonably well.

Cracking of the nipples is not uncommon in nursing mothers; perhaps half of them will develop some cracks or fissures at one time or another. There are some events which predispose the nipples to such cracking. Falling asleep while nursing may lead to maceration and cracking of the nipples; a mother should stay awake while nursing and see that the baby "attends to business." Forceably pulling the baby away from the nipple is also an occasional cause. A fissure makes nursing quite painful; this is true even when it is a hairline in width. There may occasionally be some bleeding from a crack, some of the blood being taken by the baby while nursing. If, after nursing, the baby regurgitates milk with some blood in it, the most likely source is the nipple. The cracked nipple will not heal so long as nursing is continued; hence, the baby should be promptly removed. This alone will generally lead to rapid cure.

The nipples should be protected and kept dry. Sometimes a nipple shield is recommended so as to permit continued nursing; however, the nipple may be drawn against one side of the shield and further injured. A cracked nipple may thus mean abandoning nursing; if cracking persists, a change to formula may become necessary. A heat lamp may promote healing; all that is necessary in addition is to protect the nipple with sterile gauze. (See also BREASTS.)

DAILY FOOD PATTERN FOR NURSING MOTHERS*

	Type of Food	Each Day
MILK GROUP	Milk	4-6 cups (to drink and in foods).
	Dairy products such as cheddar cheese, cottage cheese and ice cream	May sometimes be used in place of milk.
VEGETABLE-FRUIT GROUP	Select from those rich in vitamin C	2 servings.
	Grapefruit, orange, tomato (whole or as juice, canned or fresh), raw cabbage, green or sweet red pepper, broccoli, fresh strawberries, guava, mango, papaya, cantaloupe.	
	Select from those rich in vitamin A	1 or more servings.
	You can judge fairly well by color—dark green and deep yellow: apricots, broccoli, cantaloupe, carrots, greens, pumpkin, sweet potatoes, winter squash.	
	Others, including potatoes	2 or more servings.

DAILY FOOD PATTERN FOR NURSING MOTHERS* (Continued)

	Type of Food	Each Day
MEAT GROUP	Meat, poultry or fish .... Dry beans, peas, peanut butter .... Eggs	1-2 servings. Occasionally in place of meat. 1
BREAD AND CEREAL GROUP	Whole grain or enriched bread; restored breakfast cereals; and other grain products such as corn meal, grits, macaroni, spaghetti and rice	3-4 servings.
OTHER FOODS	Foods such as sugars, oils, margarine, butter, and other fats which may be used in cooking and to complete meals, provide additional food energy and other food values. Vitamin D in some form, if your food does not provide an adequate amount	According to your doctor's instructions.

89

*Reprinted from Children's Bureau Publication Number 8-1963

▶ **Involution of Uterus** After the birth of a baby the uterus begins to undergo shrinkage, a process known as involution. This process is remarkable both for the amount of shrinkage that occurs and the rapidity with which it occurs. Indeed no comparable process occurs anywhere else in the body. Within a six-week period the two-pound uterus will shrink down to two ounces. A large organ well up in the abdomen becomes a small one well down in the pelvis.

Thus, immediately after the delivery the uterus is above the level of the umbilicus (belly button). Within twenty-four hours it sinks below this level. By the fourth day after delivery it is halfway between the umbilicus and the pubic symphysis, the bony landmark felt just above the vaginal area. By the eighth day it is one-third of the way between umbilicus and symphysis, and by the tenth it has sunk below the symphysis and can no longer be felt by abdominal palpation.

During the first few days in the hospital the doctor will check on the process of involution. If it seems to be going too slowly he may prescribe medications for contracting the uterus. Nursing the infant, through an interesting tie-in between the breasts and the uterus, tends to hasten involution. It does this by increasing the contractions of the uterus, sometimes to such a point that nursing may increase afterpains. Sometimes nursing may produce a spurt in the lochia, the reddish discharge which occurs after delivery, the spurt representing increased uterine contraction. This increased vigor of the uterine contractions is desirable.

Another remarkable aspect of the involution of the uterus is that it tends to return to its old tipped-forward position in the pelvis, immediately behind the bladder. At one time it was considered that the return to this normal tipped-forward position might be aided by special exercises such as "monkey-trots," an exercise in which a woman went around on all fours for several minutes several times a day. Another procedure designed with the same end in mind was adopting the knee-chest position one or more times daily for several minutes. In this position, with the knees spread approximately eighteen inches apart, air can get into the vagina. It was felt that this might be of aid in returning the uterus to a good position. It is now generally felt, however, that the normal process of involution can be relied upon to return the structures to the usual non-pregnant state and position.

▶ **Activity After Childbirth** The amount of activity that will be permitted or encouraged during the first two weeks after delivery of the child will be dependent in part on how the pregnancy and labor went. If the labor was an easy one and not exhausting, obviously the mother will feel stronger and will be able to do more. If it was a first labor, or a difficult one perhaps associated with some blood loss and an episiotomy, the new mother can hardly be blamed for not feeling too energetic for the first day or two. She may well be advised to remain in bed during this time and use a bedpan rather than the bathroom.

However, the experience of the past twenty years has indicated that it is better for the mother to be up and about so far as possible and not to remain in bed for as long as a week or more as was formerly the practice. Muscle strength is restored earlier and activity also diminishes the possibility of clotting in the veins of the legs. In fact, if the mother has to remain in bed longer than the usual time, the doctor may well advise her to wiggle her feet at the ankles and bend them at the knees repeatedly throughout the day to stimulate the circulation. The advantages of being up and around should in no way contradict the need for rest; frequent rest periods and naps during the day are desirable.

The mother's work during delivery has correctly been called "labor," and rest is needed to accelerate the repair process. This requires mental relaxation also. A constant flow of visitors is not conducive to such relaxation, and in many maternity hospitals the number of visitors is wisely limited, sometimes to no more than two per day.

In the ordinary course of events, the average mother will be discharged around the sixth day following delivery. The return home may pose problems, since she will be faced with a great many more activities and responsibilities than existed in the hospital. In addition to running the home, there may be the needs of other family members, including perhaps other children. If this is added to the round-the-clock demands of the newborn baby, the load may be heavy indeed. A willing husband may be pressed into service, but even better is a practical nurse or a "baby nurse"—often an older woman with some experience in the field—or perhaps a mother or other close woman relative. Help of this sort will enable the mother to have adequate rest periods during the morning and the afternoon and an uninterrupted night's sleep may become possible.

For the first few days at home it may be best for her to remain on one floor if at all possible. If the home is such that it is necessary to negotiate stairs, this should be kept at a minimum. Showers and even tub baths may be permitted once a woman has returned home, but this should be checked with the doctor. If an episiotomy incision still remains open, local hot compresses or sitz baths may also be advised by the doctor. A woman can usually figure on taking short walks within a few days after she has returned home. She can be driven around in a car in about two weeks after the delivery and do the driving herself in about three to four weeks.

Soon after her return home, and perhaps even earlier if so advised, various exercises for firming up the abdomen may be advisable. Sexual relations are generally advised against until the first post-partum checkup at the doctor's office, generally at six weeks. (See SEXUAL RELATIONS AFTER CHILDBIRTH.)

▶ **Post-Partum Conditions** *Afterpains.* A fair number of women who have had more than one baby, and occasionally a woman who has had only one, may experience pains due to contractions of the uterus for several days after delivery. The pains may recur at fairly regular intervals and are more likely to be noticed if the baby is nursed. With some of these contractions, there may be an expulsion of secretion or a blood clot. The pains are sometimes sufficiently sharp to warrant taking some medication, and various pain-killing drugs will be ordered by the doctor as indicated.

Lochia. For several weeks after the delivery there is a vaginal discharge called the lochia. For the first three or four days the lochia is blood-colored, somewhat resembling a menstrual period. About the third to tenth day the discharge becomes more watery and less red in color. It then decreases in amount and may become almost colorless but will generally continue for about three weeks, when it disappears. Occasionally a slight brown discharge may persist somewhat longer. The changing appearance and amount of the lochia reflect healing changes going on within the uterus. The separation of the placenta (afterbirth) leaves a large wound surface within the uterus which contributes to the red lochia of the first days. As this area heals, the white lochia makes its appearance. The lochia has a somewhat pungent but not offensive odor; it does not ordinarily contain blood clots. It is quite normal for the amount of lochia to increase somewhat when a woman gets up and about. Sudden or unusual changes in the lochia, such as the appearance of blood clots, should be called to the doctor's attention.

Depression. "Baby blues" (post-partum depression) is a common term to describe the depressions that many women experience soon after their labor and delivery. It has been estimated that at least 60 per cent, and probably more, of new mothers experience significant depression during the first week after the delivery. Some women are ashamed to admit this and are indeed puzzled by it: the nine-month period of pregnancy has terminated successfully; the delivery has gone well; and the baby is beautiful and well-formed. What possible reason can there be for unhappiness?

Nevertheless, by about the third day following labor, a woman may find herself feeling low, lacking in energy and interest, and sometimes may burst into tears which she is unable to control. It may well be that various emotionally tinged thoughts occur to the new mother. She may feel that her having at long last fulfilled her biological role and become a mother is an important step toward aging—she is now a changed and older person. She may well also have doubts and fears about the responsibilities of motherhood and the day-in, day-out commitments this represents.

Not infrequently, however, the new mother can find no explanation to account for her tears; this in itself may add to her feelings of annoyance and depression; she merely realizes she is in the grip of an emotion she cannot readily account for and which, in fact, seems uncalled for. She should, however, be reassured that "baby blues" are very widespread in every maternity hospital; that they are generally quite temporary and almost predictably tend to disappear when the mother goes home with her new baby. There certainly is no need, nor is it advisable, to conceal her feelings. She should by all means discuss them with her doctor.

► **Post-partum Exercises** These are exercises that may be embarked on at some time shortly after the delivery, designed to hasten the return to normal strength and to the figure of the non-pregnant state. Many post-partum changes will tend to occur naturally; thus the uterus shrinks spontaneously and many varicose veins tend to diminish or disappear. The abdominal muscles, despite the considerable stretching they undergo during pregnancy—which can be the despair of a woman who prides herself on a good figure—will undergo considerable contraction once the uterus has pushed the baby into the outer world. However, what Nature will do can be helped along and somewhat improved with appropriate exercises. Not only will these exercises tighten up the abdomen, but they also tend to improve posture and are useful in the treatment of backache. The woman who is naturally the athletic sort will find them easy. If one is sedentary, do not overdo; it is better to do a small number of exercises frequently than do too large a number once or twice. Exercises can be started while in the hospital or after one returns home, as directed by the doctor. Some of them are:

1. Position: lying flat on the back. Bring right leg up eight or ten inches, let it come down slowly; repeat with the left leg, and perform this eight to ten times for each. As the days go by, one should be able to elevate each leg to approximately a right angle.

1a. After a few days this same exercise can be done with both legs. At first elevate both legs only a few inches off the bed or floor. Repeat eight to ten times. On successive days the legs can be elevated higher and higher, and lowered more and more slowly—which increases the effectiveness of the exercise. After several weeks, one should be able to bring both legs well over toward one's head. Come up and go down slowly and repeat six to ten times.

2. Position: flat on the back, arms crossed over chest. Lift the head up a few inches, then return to original position. Repeat six to ten times. As the days pass by, try raising the head higher. In four to six weeks one should be able to attain the sitting position.

3. Position: flat on the back, legs drawn up. Contract the muscles around the vaginal and rectal openings as though try-

ing to hold back a bowel movement. Repeat ten to twelve times.

4. Position: on hands and knees, weight equally distributed on all four extremities. By contracting the buttocks and stomach muscles, tilt the pelvis forward. Relax and repeat up to twelve times. This "pelvic rocking" helps relieve lumbosacral (lower back) strain.

CHOLESTEROL   Cholesterol is a wax-like member of the varied chemical family of fats. It is found in all body cells, where it is an essential structural component. In common with many other fatty substances it is constantly found circulating in the bloodstream. Here its level is remarkably constant in most individuals. The level at which it is established, however, does vary a good deal. In some families many members tend to have high blood cholesterols, a condition known as hypercholesterolemia. Similar elevations of the blood cholesterol are frequently found in diabetes and in underfunctioning of the thyroid gland, and slight rises are reported to occur under the stress of deadlines and similar pressures.

The present interest in cholesterol is based upon the fact that it has been incriminated in the process of atherosclerosis, popularly referred to as "hardening of the arteries." Cholesterol is indeed found in the fatty deposits in the arteries, although it is by no means the only fat present there. However, in a special long-term study being conducted in the population of Framingham, Mass., it has been found that elevated blood cholesterol cannot be disregarded as a factor in the background of coronary heart disease.

On the basis of such lines of evidence, certain nutritionists have advocated a reduction in the fat and cholesterol content of the American diet. Foods particularly rich in cholesterol include whole milk and its derivatives (butter, cream, most cheeses, ice cream), eggs, and the fatter cuts of meat. It is now recognized that the problem is somewhat more complicated; for in addition to the restriction of fats and cholesterol, a balance between saturated and unsaturated fats is also important (see DIET). Since cholesterol is laid down in new cells, there seems to be no reason for concern over the cholesterol intake of the growing young. Indeed, in milk and in eggs nature seems to have furnished cholesterol with this in mind.

Cholesterol must not be thought of as being all villain. In addition to being an essential part of every living cell, it is the base molecule from which the sex hormones and the hormones of the adrenal gland are formed. (See also ARTERIES, HARDENING OF.)

CIRCUMCISION   Circumcision consists of surgical removal of some of the foreskin, the excess skin which conceals the head of the penis. Sometimes the foreskin is quite tight so that it may be difficult or even impossible to pull it back. Irritation of the penis then occurs because of retained secretions (known as smegma) or even from the accumulation of small amounts of urine in this location. Circumcision performed as a religious ceremony has been practiced by the Jews and Moslems for centuries. The operation has become increasingly popular in other ethnic groups, for it has health aspects of concern to both sexes: (1) Circumcision enables the penis to be kept clean with minimal effort. (2) Irritation of the head of the penis by smegma is avoided and its sensitivity is decreased, which may be an advantage in sexual performance. (3) Cancer of the penis, although a rare disease, is even less likely to be found in a circumcised individual. (4) More importantly, cancer of the cervix (the opening of the womb) appears to have some relationship to circumcision in the male partner in the marriage. Thus cancer of the cervix is extremely rare in Jewish women; when it does occur it may well be found that the husband is not circumcised.

All the above-mentioned considerations have led to a considerable increase in the number of circumcisions. The procedure is often performed on babies within the first week or two of life, when no anesthesia is needed. In boys and men, circumcision may sometimes be necessary because the foreskin cannot be retracted, a condition called phimosis. Phimosis in babies who have not been circumcised can be prevented by pulling the foreskin back routinely whenever the baby is bathed and, if the doctor so instructs, at other times also.

COLDS, COMMON   The treatment of a common cold is generally simple. However, in a small infant, even a mild cold can make both mother and infant very uncomfortable. The child's nose is "all stopped up," which means that it is blocked with mucus. Frequently he will refuse the bottle because, as he eats with nose and mouth blocked, he has no way to get air. He therefore becomes fearful of eating.

One of the most important things in this case is to keep the nasal passages clear so he may breathe. In order to do this, the nostrils should be cleansed with cotton swabs first. You may enter the nose at least a half an inch in depth, or until resistance does not permit you to go any further. Children usually cry when this is done, not because it is painful but because it is annoying. If this mechanical cleansing of the nostrils is not effective, you should consult a doctor. He may recommend the use of a specific type of nose drop. Do not use nose drops on infants, however, unless this treatment is recommended by a doctor.

Frequently there are lumps of solid mucus in the nasal passages which block the entry of nose drops. When you place three or four drops into the nostrils and they shoot out immediately, or if they well up instead of going down into the nose, you may be sure that there is some blockage. It may be necessary to use eight or ten drops and close the infant's mouth while he is breathing *in* so that he may suck the nose drops through the nasal passage into the throat and unblock the passageway. Sometimes the drops cause him to sneeze out solid mucus. The suction apparatuses which take mucus from the nose are generally ineffective in clearing it completely. They can only reach what is in the front part of the nose. If there is blockage farther down in the passageway leading to the back of the throat, it will not be cleared. Nose drops can usually be used every three to four hours.

There are many new antihistamines with nasal decongestants which have been effective in diminishing the amount of nasal secretions. These are helpful additions in the treatment of colds and upper respiratory infections. It is usually not advisable to bathe the child when he has a cold. You may wash him off or give him a sponge bath with alcohol, or with soap and water.

Aspirin, in dosages prescribed by the doctor, can be used to reduce low-grade and higher fevers. Other medications (antibiotics) may be prescribed, not so much to cure the cold but to prevent the complications of colds, such as bronchitis and pneumonia. Cough medicines relieve cough. These should not be given unless a physician so advises.

COLITIS, FUNCTIONAL   Colitis is a general term used to refer to a large number of disorders of the colon or large intestine. Although strictly speaking *colitis,* like any medical word ending in *itis,* refers to inflammation, the term is often used to refer to disorders of motility in the large bowel without true inflammation occurring.

Disorders of functioning in the colon without inflammation are far more common than ulcerative or amebic colitis. Known as "functional colitis," the chief symptoms are either frequency of bowel movements or irregular patterns of bowel behavior in which sometimes constipation alternates with diarrhea. One pattern may consist of having two or three loose stools which may be limited only to the morning. Functional colitis is often related to stressful situations and nervous tension. Sometimes cramps and other evidences of hyperactivity of the colon are noted for which the terms "spastic colitis" or "spastic colon" are sometimes employed. Colitis is generally found in tense hypersensitive individuals, frequently of a high level of intelligence. It is felt that in these persons the large intestine is the organ that reacts to stress in a manner comparable to the organs which produce the headache or rise in blood pressure which others may experience under tension. The particular organ that thus reacts to stress is sometimes referred to as a "target organ."

Treatment. Functional colitis is treated in a variety of ways. Some of the common approaches are the following:

1. Bland diets. Most varieties of bland diets call for easily digested non-irritating types of food. Spices, condiments, alcohol, fried and greasy foods are avoided. Stimulating or laxative foods, including raw fruits and vegetables, may be restricted or omitted.

2. A variety of drugs are used to diminish hyperirritability of the colon. They may sometimes be administered in combination with tranquilizers.

3. Episodes of diarrhea may be controlled by taking paregoric or allied drugs.

4. Avoidance of tension-producing situations, a change in jobs, the talking-over of difficulties with the doctor or psychiatrist may all be useful approaches to controlling the stress that gives rise to functional colitis.

COMPRESS   A compress is a folded cloth, pad, or equivalent which can be applied to some part of the body, usually with moderate pressure. A compress may be wet or dry, hot or cold. A hot wet compress may be used to bring pimples and boils to a head, to relieve the pain of an arthritic joint, to increase the local blood supply and therefore aid bodily defenses. In many instances it will also relieve pain. A basin of hot water with two washcloths used in rotation will serve the purpose quite well.

A somewhat more convenient method is to apply the wet cloth to the area and cover it with plastic film or saran wrap. A hot-water bottle or heating pad can then be applied to maintain the heat of the compress. Care should be taken not to wet the heating pad unless it is a waterproof one. A heating pad alone is the equivalent of a hot dry compress, but for certain purposes this may not be as good as a hot wet compress. If the skin is delicate or if hot wet compresses are to be applied continuously for long periods, a prior application of cold cream or vaseline is desirable.

Cold compresses may consist of cloths wrung out of cold running water or ice water. An ice bag containing ice cubes may often conveniently serve the same purpose. Cold compresses are used for sprains and bruises, for headaches, and for relieving the discomfort of some sore throats. Paradoxically, a cold compress may sometimes serve better than a recommended hot one—for example, in bursitis, where the cold produces a numbing effect while heat, by increasing congestion, occasionally increases pain. The cold compress can be applied for five to fifteen minutes or even longer; if, however, it produces uncomfortable sensations of cold, it should be used in an on-and-off manner: for example, five minutes on and five minutes off.

The immediate effect of cold applications on sprains or bruises is to cut down pain and swelling, and to diminish any bleeding that may result from the injury. Often within the first twelve to twenty-four hours cold compresses are advocated, which are then to be followed by heat. Thus, after removal of a tooth or other dental manipulation, the immediate application of cold will diminish swelling and pain; application of heat the following day will promote the rate of healing.

CONCUSSION   A fall or the impact of a blow to the head may produce an injury which results in a brief loss of consciousness. This is referred to as a concussion. Sometimes the victim appears dazed after he recovers, may be confused as to the events that led to the injury or have a loss of memory in relation to events for some longer period of time prior to the injury. There are all degrees of concussion—from relatively brief losses of consciousness with virtually no aftereffect, on to more prolonged episodes with greater memory damage. Some of the latter are followed by what is known as the post-concussive syndrome, in which the individual complains of recurrent headaches, feelings of faintness, or other symptoms.

Fortunately the brain receives excellent protection from the fluid immediately surrounding it and the sturdy box we call the skull. Most bumps on the head will not affect it at all. Occasionally, however, bleeding may occur from one of the blood vessels within the skull. There may be a brief period of unconsciousness, often regarded as a concussion, from which the person recovers. After a variable period during which he appears conscious or perhaps somewhat dazed, the victim may lapse into unconsciousness again. This sequence is generally due to bleeding within the skull, a common form of which is known as subdural hematoma. It will need prompt medical attention.

CONGENITAL DISORDERS

▶ **Congenital Megacolon** This is a disorder due to a defect in the nerve cells of the rectosigmoid portion of the intestines which results in an absence of normal bowel movements. Stool accumulates and cannot be pushed out. This causes progressive constipation with enlargement of the colon and abdomen. It usually begins in early infancy and is characterized by passage of stool every four to five days.

The treatment of this condition is surgical. The disordered section of bowel is eliminated, and the condition cured.

► **Phenylketonuria (PKU)** Phenylketonuria is an inherited protein disorder of the metabolism transmitted by an autosomal recessive gene. If a family has one child with this disease, the chance of a second occurring is one in four, or 25 per cent. Although PKU occurs frequently (one in every 40,000 babies in the United States), it is treatable. Untreated cases account for 1 per cent of the institutionalized mental defectives. PKU is caused by lack of the liver enzyme *phenylalanine hydroxylase* which converts phenylalanine to tyrosine. Excessive accumulation of L-phenylalanine in the blood, eventually excreted in the urine as phenylacetyl glutamine, accounts for the typical mousy, musty odor of the baby's urine.

Children with PKU may appear normal at birth. They frequently are blond with blue eyes, and suffer from eczema. They fail to develop mentally and often show epileptic seizures and an abnormal electroencephalogram. Diagnosis is made by testing the suspected urine for phenylpyruvic acid with a specially prepared piece of filter paper. Chemical tests for measuring phenylalanine blood levels confirm the diagnosis.

Treatment is with a diet low in phenylalanine. In general, children treated early enough (before six months of age) have a better chance of avoiding severe retardation. Treatment before two years of age results in children who are educable but mentally handicapped. A child over two years of age may be too retarded to train, although there are isolated cases of untreated phenylketonurics who are of average intelligence. Many hospitals now have a screening process for PKU in newborn infants.

► **Pyloric Stenosis** Infants with this disease are born with it (congenital). Pyloric stenosis is a thickening of the muscle around the duodenum where the stomach enters the intestines. Occurring mostly in boys, the main symptom is projectile vomiting of all foods before seven or eight weeks of age. The child is normally hungry and has a good appetite, but after swallowing a few ounces of milk, shoots it out immediately. Most normal babies do spit up a small amount when they are burped, when the stomach is compressed, or if they are placed on their stomachs after a feeding.

Mechanical pressure will cause some spitting up. However, the type of vomiting seen in pyloric stenosis is persistent and unremitting. There is never any bile in the vomit, indicating that the vomiting comes from an obstructed area above the bile-duct entrance into the intestines. The infant becomes constipated and loses weight. Frequently a small, olive-size tumor mass may be felt in the child's abdomen. He may become dehydrated due to fluid loss from vomiting. Corrective treatment is usually surgical if medical management fails.

CONSTIPATION Constipation should be regarded as the passage of hard, dried, or pellety stools rather than the failure to have regular or daily bowel movements. Thus, constipation can exist even in the presence of daily movements. Since a good deal of the bulk of the stool is its water content, people who are constipated generally complain that the stools are smaller. They sometimes regard this as evidence that they are retaining wastes, which is an erroneous supposition. Many of the ills ascribed to constipation are exaggerated; some individuals, however, do experience mild headache, a sub-par feeling, abdominal distention, and "gas." Symptoms end with a satisfactory evacuation.

Constipation is quite common during pregnancy, in part because the intestinal musculature seems to be relaxed and because the enlarged uterus may exert pressure against the lower part of the large intestine.

Treatment. There are several measures that may be helpful:

1. Sipping a cup of hot water the first thing in the morning.
2. Increasing the amount of fruits and fruit juices in the diet—particularly prunes, prune juice, figs, apples. Salads and green leafy vegetables are bulk stimulants.
3. Consumption of six to eight glasses of water daily.
4. Possible use of mineral oil, stool softeners, and other laxatives (see DRUGS AND REMEDIES).
5. Glycerine or Ducolax® suppositories, or prepackaged enemas containing sodium phosphate (Fleet enema, Travad enema) act within a few minutes to relieve constipation.

Your doctor may have other suggestions and diets that may be of use. In general, constipation that comes on with pregnancy promptly disappears after the delivery. Admittedly also, constipation becomes more of a problem in the later years and is a common complaint in the older age groups. Any of the measures mentioned above may be applicable. (See CONGENITAL DISORDERS—Congenital Megacolon.)

CONVULSIONS   Convulsions, commonly called "fits" or seizures, are caused by many different conditions. The eyes roll up into the head, the jaws are clamped shut, and one loses consciousness as the body stiffens. Parts of the body then shake with twitching or convulsive movements. There may be difficulty in breathing, and the color of the skin may change to reddish purple or bluish. There may be some frothing at the mouth. Sometimes high fever or the onset of some illness may cause a convulsion. More serious causes of convulsions are brain disorders (epilepsy, brain tumors) and poisoning. Most convulsions are self-limited: one may be unconscious for one or two minutes, then come around.

When there is a convulsive seizure there is also spasm of the throat muscles. Grinding motions may injure the tongue; later, the tongue may fall back into the throat; nasal and respiratory passages fill with mucus. It is important to pry open the teeth with a wooden or metal tool (the handle of a knife or a spoon) and draw the tongue forward. It can be held with a towel—this will guard against choking. The mucus may be wiped from the back of the mouth and, if possible, mouth-to-mouth resuscitation performed. If there is any rubber tubing handy, it can be inserted into the nose or mouth, and with suction much of the mucus may be removed. This is an emergency measure which permits air to enter.

In many cities an emergency oxygen service exists as part of the police department. A call to the police will often bring the emergency squad to administer oxygen to a convulsing person. The victim should be placed in a lukewarm bath until help arrives, making sure, of course, that his nose and mouth are kept out of the water. This will often relax him and stop the convulsion.

Hospitalization is important after a convulsive seizure to determine its cause. It will also ensure proper treatment in case one convulsion is followed by a second.

CORONARY THROMBOSIS   The coronary arteries are the main channels which conduct blood to the heart. Formation of a clot within the vessel, known as a thrombosis, will cut off the circulation to a portion of heart muscle. As a consequence the muscle tissue dies off and is replaced by scar tissue. Such a clot never forms in a normal artery and is most commonly seen in arteries in which the fat depositions of atherosclerosis have previously occurred.

Coronary thrombosis is associated with severe pain, usually felt under the breast bone, which commonly radiates to the arms or to the neck. The pain may last for hours and require narcotics for relief. Various disorders of the heart rate and of the circulation may accompany this, one of the more critical ones being a severe drop in blood pressure with a shock-like state. This may require the emergency use of special drugs designed to raise blood pressure. Occasionally the symptoms are less marked, or they may be referred to the digestive tract, with symptoms such as nausea and vomiting perhaps secondary to congestion there. Or acute congestion may occur in the lungs, producing marked shortness of breath.

Once the acute symptoms have been treated, an enforced rest will be the next step. It is known that it takes at least three to four weeks for a firm scar to form within the damaged heart muscle. During this time the patient may be kept in bed, although some physicians may permit him to sit in a bedside chair for parts of the day. Anticoagulant drugs, which diminish the rate of clot formation of the blood, may be given to the patient with a coronary thrombosis, and may even be kept up for months afterwards. There are some risks inherent in this method of treatment, and not all physicians subscribe to the benefits to be derived therefrom.

With current methods of treatment, the great majority of victims of a coronary thrombosis recover and can be expected to resume usual activities. In some instances the impaired efficiency of the heart as a pump may necessarily lead to restriction of physical activities. In recent years the use of diets emphasizing polyunsaturated fats for victims of coronary thrombosis has been advocated by the American Heart Association.

Up until about the age of fifty, heart attacks are a good deal more common in men than in women. Thereafter the coronary thrombosis rate begins to rise in women, and at sixty and beyond the rate in women approximates that in men. It has therefore been concluded that the female sex hormone produced by a woman's ovaries protects her against coronary thrombosis and other vascular disorders but that the protection disappears after the menopause. (See also ARTERIES, HARDEN-ING OF.)

CRAMPS AND COLIC

► **Cramps** Cramps are painful contractions of muscles. They may occur either in the voluntary muscles, those we use in movement, or the involuntary muscles, sometimes called smooth muscles. (The latter are found in such internal organs as the uterus, urinary bladder, and gallbladder and in the stomach and intestines.)

Muscular cramps occur most frequently in the legs, often at night when they produce awakening from sleep. They are com-plained of by young individuals with good circulatory systems and hence are not necessarily a sign of a poor circulation. They are also a fairly frequent complaint during pregnancy where possibly they are related to the pressure of the enlarg-ing uterus on the great veins running up from the extremities. Various drugs are used for leg cramps, including large doses of calcium and tranquilizers with muscle-relaxing properties. At times nothing works too well and the only relief may be se-cured by getting out of bed and walking about briefly.

"Abdominal cramps" is a general term applied to recurrent pains arising in the digestive tract or in an associated organ. They are sometimes referred to as "colicky pains" and typically come in waves, rise to a certain level, then decrease until the next wave of contractions begins. Various kinds of inflamma-tions, the passage of stones, toxins, or irritants may all be causative. Many of the factors that lead to vomiting will pro-duce crampy pains in the upper abdomen, and similarly the many causes of diarrhea will set up colicky pains in the large intestine. Consultation with the doctor, and sometimes X-rays or other procedures, may be indicated.

► **Colic of Early Infancy** Colic is a condition of painful ab-dominal cramps. It is produced by many different conditions occurring in the first three to six months of life. It may be caused by hunger or distention of the abdomen from swallow-ing too much air ("gas pains"). Infants get red in the face, draw their legs up and cry with extreme pain. If the infant is able to burp the gas, or pass it through the rectum, he is gen-erally relieved and the crying stops.

Overfeeding (too many ounces of milk, or too rich a formula) may cause colic. Allergies to certain milks may cause colicky pains. There may also be mechanical causes: for example, a nipple which does not have holes adequate to permit enough milk to come through will cause the infant to suck mostly air (and gas). He will not really be properly nourished, and the air or gas cause distention and pain.

Treatment. The treatment of colic depends on the cause. If the child is allergic, is on a heavy formula which disagrees with him, or is taking solid foods too early, obviously the elimination of the causes will relieve the cramps. There are also some symptomatic measures which will relieve the pain, such as a hot-water bottle applied to the abdomen, sedatives, and antispasmodics. Frequently burping in order to get the gas up will be helpful, as will warm baths. Introduction of an enema bone to help the child pass gas through the rectum may relieve the pain. Usually colic subsides after the first three or four months.

CYSTIC FIBROSIS   Cystic fibrosis of the pancreas combines a fat and starch deficiency with a defect in the mucus-secreting glands of the entire body. It is an inborn error of metabolism affecting the exocrine glands, such as the mucus, sweat, and salivary glands. The affected glands produce an abnormally thick and tenacious mucus which in turn produces lung, pancreas, and liver changes by obstructing the flow of air and fluid in these organs. The sweat glands secrete abnormally increased amounts of sodium and chloride (salt).

Chronic respiratory disease is the most prominent part of cystic fibrosis. Bronchial mucus obstruction predisposes to recurring infections with progressive damage to lung tissue. The insufficiency of pancreatic trypsin, lipase, and amylase (pancreatic enzymes) causes intestinal malabsorption. The stools are malodorous, greasy, and bulky in spite of a normal food intake. A very reliable diagnostic test in these infants, if they are over six weeks of age, is the sweat electrolyte test. Infants with this disease show increased excretion of sodium, chloride, and potassium in their perspiration. The test is made by placing a hand print on an agar plate. The sweat chlorides react with the silver nitrate and potassium chromate in the agar, producing a positive test. Other tests to confirm the diagnosis examine duodenal enzymes and mucus secretions.

Treatment. Treatment of cystic fibrosis is a high calorie, high protein, and low fat diet. Pancreatic extracts have to be given in addition. The frequent respiratory infections must be prevented and treated immediately when they do occur. Children with cystic fibrosis are particularly liable to heat prostration in summer due to abnormal loss of salts in their sweat. They may develop severe crises of shock and dehydration.

DIABETES MELLITUS   Diabetes mellitus is a disorder of carbohydrate metabolism. It is rare in early childhood. Approximately 10 per cent of the cases begin before fifteen years of age, and are usually inherited. There are associated abnormalities in fat and protein metabolism producing high amounts of sugar in the blood and urine.

The exact cause is not known. However, the following facts are important in the development of the disease: Insulin, the important secretion of the pancreas, is necessary for the storage of glycogen (sugar) in the liver. If insulin is not produced, no glycogen can be stored, consequently the body burns fat and protein instead, at a very high rate. Metabolism of fat and protein produces ketone bodies which cannot be excreted in the urine and cannot be further metabolized by muscles. They accumulate in the blood and cause acidosis. In order to remove these organic acids through the bloodstream, base (substance reacting with acid to produce salt and water) is lost by the kidney, thus increasing the degree of acidosis. Large amounts of water are necessary for the kidneys to excrete the sugar and acid products. This leads to dehydration. Symptoms of thirst and excess excretion of water occur.

Symptoms. The classical symptoms of diabetes, therefore, are: polyuria (excessive urination), polyphagia (excessive eating), and polydipsia (excessive drinking). Weight is lost in spite of adequate eating. Diabetics show unusually high levels of sugar in both bloodstream and urine. The glucose tolerance test which is specific for diabetes shows a blood sugar curve rising above normal levels and a slower return to fasting levels. The blood cholesterol and fat levels in many cases are high, and there may be chemical findings of acidosis.

Treatment. The treatment of diabetes is replacement with insulin. The insulin metabolizes the glucose from the blood stream and prevents the formation of ketone bodies. There are many different forms of insulin. Protamine zinc insulin acts over a period of twenty-four to forty-eight hours. Diet and calorie control are important in the treatment of diabetes, particularly in children. In infants of "uncontrolled" diabetic mothers, a condition of temporary hyperinsulism resulting in low blood sugar may occur.

Several new pills have been developed which can be taken by mouth and effectively lower the blood sugar. However, these have not been effective in the treatment of children, and therefore *they* must still take their insulin by injection. With treatment and proper medication, diabetes can be maintained under reasonable control.

Diabetic children are particularly susceptible to infections. Any child who is diabetic and has fever with infection should be carefully supervised by a physician. Diabetic coma and insulin shock are major problems in the management of diabetic children. The symptoms of insulin shock (too much insulin) are: tingling sensations, sweating, irritability, pallor, followed by delirium, unconsciousness, and convulsions. It is treated by giving sugar immediately either by mouth or injection.

Diabetic coma is characterized by apathy, drowsiness, restlessness, and deep rapid breathing. The skin is dry, the lips cherry red, and the breath may have a fruity (acetone) odor. Vomiting and headache may occur. Treatment is insulin.

DIAGNOSTIC PROCEDURES

► **Cystoscopy** This is a procedure through which the bladder is visualized by passing an instrument (cystoscope) up the urethra (urinary channel) and thus into the bladder. The instrument has a lens system and a special bulb at the tip which furnishes light. Infection, tumors, stones may be directly observed.

► **Proctoscopy** Here a similar but larger instrument is passed into the rectal region, thus permitting direct inspection to a level as high as six or seven inches.

► **Electrocardiograph (ECG)** This is an instrument which picks up the electrical currents generated by the beating heart, amplifies them. and transmits them to a moving stylus. A tracing is inscribed which may reveal abnormalities such as irregularities (arrhythmias), or areas of damage such as result from a coronary attack.

▶ **Electroencephalogram (EEG)** This is a similar instrument which records brain waves. It is of help in diagnosing various forms of epilepsy, brain tumors, damage produced by circulatory changes, etc.

DIAPERS, CARE OF A baby may use up to a dozen or more diapers a day, depending on how much he is awake. Diapers need to be soft, light in weight, and not clumsy. The material they are made of should soak up moisture well, wash easily, and dry fast. Those made of birdseye or of knit goods are much used. Gauze diapers absorb moisture well·and dry very fast. They are made of two thin layers woven together at the edges instead of hemmed. They wear as well as those of heavier material.

Unless waterproof diaper covers are loose, and are cut so that the air can circulate, they may be uncomfortably warm or cause a rash on the baby's buttocks. Some babies are able to wear them much of the time with no harmful effects whatever. Instead of using waterproof pants, some mothers cut a piece of plastic material into 8- by 10-inch squares that fit between the folds of the diaper and do not touch the baby's skin.

As your baby gets older and takes larger amounts of liquid, you may find he gets so wet at night that you feel he will be more comfortable with a waterproof diaper cover that keeps his bed from getting wet and chilly. Try out moisture-proof pants for overnight use. You can soon tell whether your baby is one of those whose skin is too sensitive to make their use safe for hours at a time.

When you wash the diapers at home put them to soak in a covered pail of cold water as soon as you take them off the baby. If the diaper is soiled, shake or scrape off as much as you can of the stool, and rub a little soap into the stained parts before putting it to soak. To wash diapers use any mild soap, soap powder, or detergent in plenty of hot water. The rinsing is just as important as the washing, for unless you get all the soap out, the baby's tender skin is liable to become irritated. If the water in your locality is soft, two or three rinsings may be enough. With hard water, three or four rinsings are usually necessary to completely rid the diapers of soap. It is all right to use a little bleach in the wash water if you put the diapers through several rinse waters. If you can dry diapers outdoors, the sunlight will take out most stains. It is usually unnecessary to boil diapers if they are thoroughly washed and rinsed. They are softer if dried outdoors, and bacteria have little chance of remaining in diapers dried in the sun.

If your baby has a tender skin that makes him get diaper rash easily, you will need to use special care to keep him free of the irritation caused by wet diapers. You can prevent the ammonia odor in wet diapers and protect your baby's skin either by boiling the diapers, ironing them with a hot iron, or by putting in the last rinse water some product your doctor suggests.

A baby whose diapers are free of soap and are changed promptly is quite unlikely to have much, if any, trouble with diaper rash. But if your baby's buttocks tend to break out with a rash very easily, you may feel that boiling or ironing his diapers is a small price to pay for his comfort. Leaving off a baby's diaper and exposing his skin to the sun and air or to the warmth of an electric light helps to do away with diaper rash. If an electric light is used, be sure that it is at a safe distance from the baby, so that he cannot be burned.

DIARRHEA AND DYSENTERY   There are many causes for diarrhea, ranging from spoiled or laxative foods, emotional upsets and tensions, to a group of inflammations of the colon produced by various organisms. The latter are frequently referred to as dysentery. It is not always easy to distinguish among these causes: thus the symptoms of a viral diarrhea and a mild food poisoning might be quite indistinguishable, with cramps, frequency of bowel movement, perhaps with little or no fever. Both types of disorders might respond equally to a bland diet, antispasmodic drugs, paregoric, perhaps also to a heating pad applied to the abdomen.

Viral dysentery is the mildest form of dysentery. It is often seen in epidemics, particularly during the winter and spring.

Although it may produce severe abdominal pains, more often the cramps are relatively mild. This diarrhea seldom lasts more than a few days and there is no bloody mucus in the bowel movements.

Bacillary dysenteries generally produce frequent odorous stools and often contain pus and blood. Within a day or so the colon usually has emptied itself and the stools that are passed consist largely of mucus. For bacillary dysenteries the physician will prescribe antibiotics or certain drugs of the sulfonamide group.

Amebic dysentery is uncommon in the United States. The diagnosis can be made by examining a portion of freshly passed stool under the microscope. Several of the antibiotics, or Atabrine® (a drug used in malaria) and Carbarsone® (an arsenical drug), are useful in the treatment of amebic dysenteries.

Most of the simple diarrheas are more of a nuisance than a threat, although in infants the loss of large amounts of fluid may produce a grave situation and call for emergency measures. Consult your doctor immediately.

In older age groups it is traditional to limit the diet to such foods as tea and toast, and binding foods such as farina, oatmeal, tapioca, and mashed potatoes. Later, relatively bland and digestible foods are added, such as chicken, eggs, fish, and broiled meats. Kaopectate®, a suspension of kaolin in pectin, and paregoric are frequently employed. Certain drugs that relax the large bowel and diminish its activity, known as antispasmodics, may also be prescribed. Some of the weakness produced by diarrhea is due to the loss of salts, particularly sodium and potassium, from the body. Non-laxative fruit juices such as apple juice or tomato juice, to which a sprinkle of salt has been added, will be useful in compensating for these lost salts.

DIET, CALCIUM REQUIREMENTS   Calcium is a widely distributed and basic mineral found in the blood and in all the tissues. It is the chief mineral that goes into the structure of bones. Calcium is involved in the formation of blood clots, and it regulates the performance of muscle tissue. Dietary calcium is of particular concern to women because of the increased need for it during pregnancy and during lactation (nursing). Every mother should also know that the calcium needs of her children are considerably higher than those of the adult because of bone growth. Even after the period of reproduction and child-rearing has ended, calcium still continues to be of concern.

At least 20 per cent of the women of the United States will develop osteoporosis, a condition in which the bones become brittle. (This accounts for the frequency of fractures in aging women.) Nutritional studies indicate that many adults as well as adolescents fail to get recommended daily allotments of calcium. In three out of ten households the average diet contains less than the recommended amounts of calcium; in fact, of all the nutrients we eat calcium is most likely to be lacking. Recommended daily allowances for calcium are as follows:

Adults, all ages and sexes—0.8 gm.
Women, pregnant (second half)—1.5 gm.
Women, nursing—2.0 gm.
Children, 1 to 10—1.0 gm.
Teenagers, 13 to 19—1.3-1.4 gm.

From a practical point of view it is difficult to get enough calcium without drinking milk, one quart of which will supply 1 gm. Two cups of milk will thus supply about ¾ of the adult's daily requirement. For those who worry about calories, skimmed milk has the same calcium value as whole milk. A pregnant woman should probably drink at least one quart of milk per day, a nursing mother a quart and a half.

Other good sources of calcium are some of the cheeses, but this is variable. Swiss and cheddar cheese contain about 250 mg., (¼ gm.), in a one-ounce portion, but one ounce of cottage cheese contains only 25 mg. and cream cheese only 18. A medium serving of ice cream has about 115 mg. Vegetables and fruits are the next best source of calcium. One cupful of most vegetables furnishes 35 to 70 mg. Vegetables particularly rich in calcium are broccoli, kale, collards, and turnip and mustard greens. Whole wheat flour contains two or three times the calcium of white flour.

DIET, CRASH AND FORMULA   These are nutritionally restricted diets which can be embarked upon for only a few days, and with which a daily multiple vitamin supplement is necessary. Crash diets may produce an encouraging weight loss and enable one to go on to a more orthodox reducing diet. Examples of crash diets applicable to both lunch and dinner are: (1) One or two bananas plus a glass of skimmed milk. (2) Three-fourths cup of cottage cheese plus a glass of skimmed milk. (3) One or two hard-boiled eggs plus one quarter head of lettuce sprinkled with lemon juice and a glass of skimmed milk. In addition, chewing raw celery or carrots for between-meal hunger is permitted.

Formula diets, such as Metrecal® or equivalents, generally consist of skimmed-milk products to which vitamins and sometimes oils are added. A typical portion contains 225 calories, and if unsweetened tea or coffee are taken in addition, three or four meals would amount to 675 to 900 calories per day. The formula diets work, at least initially, because of their restriction in calories and the fact that no choice is permitted. Also, the oil that some of the products contain leads to a feeling of satiety. Some digestive disturbances may be encountered because of the oil, however.

Appetite-curbing drugs, many of which are derived from the amphetamine family, enable some people markedly to reduce their calorie intake without feeling hungry or having such symptoms as weakness or faintness.

For individuals with low basal metabolism, thyroid is sometimes prescribed as part of a weight-loss program. Also, if there are evidences of fluid retention on a reduction program, a pill to produce loss of water (a diuretic) may be prescribed. Obviously drugs in any of these classes can be taken only under a doctor's supervision. (See also DIET, REDUCING.)

DIET, FOOD GUIDE   The U.S. Department of Agriculture has developed a simplified and basic approach to healthful eating. It is based on sound findings developed by nutritional scientists and is sometimes known as the basic food guide. Nutritionists everywhere use it as a base for the developments of all kinds of special diets. Whether a diet is low in calories, high or low in salt, or has other special features, one is likely to find the basic food guide forming its foundation. It consists of the following four groups:

1. MILK GROUP. The following amounts of milk should be used daily: Children, 3 to 4 glasses; teenagers, 4 or more

glasses; adults, **2** or more glasses; mothers-to-be, **4** or more; nursing mothers, at least **6** glasses. Cheese, ice cream, and other milk-derived foods can supply part of the daily milk requirement. In terms of the calcium content in milk, count one slice of cheese (1 ounce) as 2/3 glass of milk, ½ cup of cottage cheese as 1/3 glass, ¼ pint of ice cream as ¼ glass of milk.

2. MEAT GROUP. Two or more servings daily of beef, veal, pork, lamb, poultry, fish, or eggs. Dried beans, peas, and nuts may be used as occasional alternatives. A serving is 2 to 3 ounces (without bone) of lean cooked meat, poultry, or fish (1 slice or 2 thin slices); 2 eggs; 1 cup of cooked dried beans, dried peas, or lentils; 4 tablespoons of peanut butter.

3. VEGETABLE-FRUIT GROUP. Four or more servings daily. Include a citrus fruit or other source of vitamin C and also a dark green or deep yellow vegetable for vitamin A at least every other day. Other vegetables and fruits can make up the suggested servings. A serving consists of ½ cup of vegetable or fruit, or a portion ordinarily served, such as a medium-sized apple, banana, orange, or half a medium-sized grapefruit or cantaloupe.

Vitamin C Group. Fruit and vegetables important for vitamin C include oranges and grapefruit and their juices, cantaloupe, fresh strawberries, broccoli, and peppers. Less rich sources of vitamin C, two servings of which equal one serving of the above, include: asparagus tips, Brussels sprouts, cabbage, collards, garden cress, kale, kohlrabi, mustard greens, potatoes or sweet potatoes cooked in their jackets, spinach, tomatoes and tomato juice, and turnip greens. Other fruits include honeydew melon, tangerine, tangerine juice, lemons and lemon juice, and watermelon.

Vegetables for Vitamin A. Broccoli, carrots, chard, collards, cress, kale, spinach, turnip greens, and other dark green leaves, sweet potatoes, pumpkin, or winter squash. (Apricots and cantaloupe can also serve as a source of vitamin A.)

4. BREAD-CEREAL GROUP. Four or more servings daily of the whole grain, enriched or restored kinds. (Check the label to be sure that they are "enriched.") A serving consists of one slice of bread, 1 ounce of ready-to-eat cereal, ½ to ¾ cup of cooked cereal, corn meal, grits, macaroni, noodles, rice, or spaghetti.

114

DIET, PRUDENT The Bureau of Nutrition of New York City's Department of Health has developed a dietary program referred to as the Prudent Diet, which emphasizes the unsaturated fats. There is evidence that individuals who have had a heart attack are less likely to have a second one if they follow this diet; at present it would also seem reasonable to eat in this way to avoid having heart attacks or other forms of hardening of the arteries. The Prudent Diet emphasizes substantial cuts in most meats, eggs, whole milk, whole-milk cheeses, sweet and sour cream, ice cream, butter, etc. The following are the highlights of the program:

1. FISH, MEAT, EGGS. Fish and shell fish at least four to five times a week, for any meal. The fat in fish is an excellent source of polyunsaturated fatty acids. Poultry may be taken often; it is low in fat. Veal may be taken frequently—it is a lean meat; beef, pork, and lamb not more than three to four times a week, with the serving not to exceed four ounces of cooked meat. Eggs, not more than four a week for adults; four to seven a week for children. Avoid very fat meats, bacon, sausage, corned beef, pastrami. Select lean cuts of all meats. Trim off all visible fat. Keep portions moderate—four to six ounces before cooking (four ounces after cooking).

2. MILK AND MILK PRODUCTS. The fat in whole milk is predominantly saturated and is not recommended. Two cups of skimmed milk daily for adults—two to four cups of milk daily for children; two cups of this milk allowance may be whole milk. More than four cups of milk are not recommended for children, even for adolescents. Cottage, pot, or farmer cheese often. Avoid butter, cream, ice cream, cream cheese, hard cheeses, and other whole-milk cheeses.

3. FATS. Vegetable oils should be used for their polyunsaturated fatty acids. To have more of these than saturated fatty acids, use vegetable oils daily. Use 1½ ounces (3 tablespoons) daily in cooking and at table. Make salad dressings with oil. Substitute oil for other fats in cooking and baking. Butter, ordinary margarine, and other hydrogenated fats must be kept at a minimum.

DIET, REDUCING There is no satisfactory long-term answer to overweight that does not call for some self-discipline. Losing weight, however rapidly, only to regain it however slowly or rapidly, only leads to cycles of self-torture and aggravation which in the long run may be hardly worthwhile. It is better to find a more stable solution, whether this means giving up rich desserts, bread, carbonated sweet beverages and candy, or increasing one's exercise. Among the dietary programs that may be applicable are:

1. A HIGH-PROTEIN REDUCING DIET. The program focuses on a small-to-moderate-sized portion of meat, poultry, or fish for both lunch and dinner. To this is added a salad with a low-calorie dressing and 5 per cent vegetables, such as string beans, asparagus, broccoli, zucchini, etc. No bread, rolls, or sweet desserts are permitted, though half of a grapefruit or cantaloupe, or their equivalent, can be included. Two cups of skimmed milk per day may be taken, and can be used for the mid-afternoon snack, or before retiring. The success of this diet is dependent on the high-satiety value of meats.

2. BALANCED LOW-CALORIE DIETS. These are diets in which the various food items normally consumed are represented, but are selected as to quantity (smaller portions), or as to quality (low as against high-calorie desserts, 5 per cent vegetables as against 15 per cent vegetables, etc.). It is seldom practicable to reduce the total calorie intake of the day below 1000 calories. Numerous diets are available in which the calories are totaled up, but rather than following them rigidly it is probably better to grasp their essence and follow the principles. Instead of bacon, eggs, butter, and cream in the course of the morning breakfast, one would have juice, a small portion of a dry cereal with skimmed milk, and coffee with a little whole milk. For lunch and supper one could choose from a protein, such as listed above, a scoop of cottage cheese, or one to two eggs, to which will be added a salad or 5 per cent vegetable, 1 slice of bread, and a fruit or other low-calorie dessert. Contrast for example pie (350 calories) or ice cream (250 calories) with half a grapefruit (50 calories) or half a cantaloupe (40 calories), a tangerine (40 calories), or an apple (70 calories).

DIET, REDUCING
► First Day
LOW CALORIE—1,200 Calories
BREAKFAST

Grapefruit .... ½ medium

Wheat flakes ....1 ounce
Skim milk ....1½ cups
Coffee (black), if desired.

LUNCH

Chef's salad:
Julienne chicken ....1 ounce
Cheddar cheese ....½ ounce
Hard-cooked egg ....½ egg
Tomato ....1 large
Cucumber ....6 slices
Endive ....½ ounce
Lettuce ....⅛ head
French dressing ....2 tablespoons
Rye wafers ....4 wafers
Skim milk ....1 cup

DINNER

Beef pot roast ....3 ounces
Mashed potatoes ....⅓ cup
Green peas ....½ cup
Whole-wheat bread ....1 slice
Butter or margarine ....½ teaspoon
Fruit cup:
Orange ....½ small
Apple ....½ small
Banana ....½ medium

► Second Day

BREAKFAST

Orange juice ....½ cup
Soft-cooked egg ....1 egg
Whole-wheat toast ....1 slice
Butter or margarine ....1 teaspoon
Skim milk ....1 cup
Coffee (black), if desired.

LUNCH

Sandwich:
Enriched bread ....2 slices
Boiled ham ....1½ ounces
Mayonnaise ....2 teaspoons

Mustard
Lettuce ....1 large leaf
Celery ....1 small stalk
Radishes ....4 radishes
Dill pickle ....½ large
Skim milk ....1 cup

DINNER

Roast lamb ....3 ounces
Rice, converted ....½ cup
Spinach ....¾ cup
Lemon ....¼ medium
Salad:
    Peaches, canned ....1 peach half
    Cottage cheese ....⅓ cup
    Lettuce ....1 large leaf

BETWEEN-MEAL SNACK

Apple ....1 medium

► Third Day

BREAKFAST

Tomato juice ....½ cup
French toast:
    Enriched bread ....1 slice
    Egg ....½ egg
    Milk
Butter or margarine ....1 teaspoon
Jelly ....1½ teaspoons
Skim milk ....1 cup
Coffee (black) if desired.

LUNCH

Tunafish salad:
    Tunafish ....2 ounces
    Hard-cooked egg ....½ egg
    Celery ....1 small stalk
    Lemon juice ....1 teaspoon
    Salad dressing ....1½ tablespoons
    Lettuce ....1 large leaf
Whole-wheat bread ....2 slices

Butter or margarine .... 1 teaspoon
Carrot sticks .... ½ carrot
Skim milk .... 1 cup

DINNER

Beef liver .... 3 ounces
Green snap beans .... ⅔ cup
Shredded cabbage .... ⅔ cup
with vinegar dressing.
Roll, enriched .... 1 small
Butter or margarine .... ½ teaspoon
Grapes .... 1 small bunch

BETWEEN-MEAL SNACK

Orange .... 1 medium

DIET REQUIREMENTS IN CHILDHOOD— MALNUTRITION

▶ **Caloric Requirements** *Infants:* 45 to 55 calories per pound of expected body weight and for age of the child.

Children: 1,000 calories basic plus 100 calories for each year. Example: an eight-year-old child should have 1,000 plus 800, or 1,800 calories per day.

▶ **Protein Requirements** *Infants:* 2 grams per pound of body weight. Thus if a child takes one and three-quarter ounces of whole milk per pound per day, or a little less than one ounce of evaporated milk per pound per day, this will assure adequate protein intake.

Children: 1 gram per pound of body weight until the age of eleven or twelve. Later, slightly more is required. If approximately 20 per cent of the required calorie intake is protein, this will be adequate.

▶ **Minerals (Daily Requirements)**
Calcium: 1 to 1.5 grams
Phosphorous: 1.5 grams
Iron: 16 milligrams
Iodine: 100 to 200 micrograms

The following daily diet composition will satisfy basic growth needs:

Milk: ¾ to 1 quart
Meat, poultry or fish: 1 serving (5 or 6 weekly)

Liver: 1 serving weekly

Eggs: 1 (5 or 6 weekly)

Vegetables: 1 raw, 1 pigmented—2 servings daily

Fruit, fresh: 1 citrus—2 or more servings daily

Butter: 2 teaspoons daily

Bread, enriched or whole grain, and cereals: enough to meet caloric needs

Cod liver oil: 1 teaspoon or equivalent in multiple vitamins daily.

► **Malnutrition** This refers to a state of poor nutrition which may be caused by inadequate vitamin intake (leading to rickets or scurvy) or inadequate intake of specific nutritional elements. Inadequate calorie or protein intake will result in different forms of diseases.

Symptoms. Failure to gain weight and progressive emaciation occur. The abdomen may be distended, and the infant may take on the appearance of a withered old man. Specific vitamin deficiencies will produce evidence of rickets, scurvy, beriberi, pellagra, and other conditions. Protein deficiency produces kwashiorkor. In this condition there may be pot belly, skin rash, and hair color changes; the hair frequently falls out.

Chronically malnourished children may not necessarily be underweight. They may show increased susceptibility to infection, pale skin, muddy complexion, poor teeth, delayed bone development, and may find it difficult to pay attention in school. Fatigue, restlessness, and nervousness are common.

Treatment. Preventive treatment is accomplished by providing a diet adequate in calorie, protein, fat, carbohydrate, and vitamin content. Treatment of malnutrition, once it has been established, is directed towards providing an adequate diet containing all the above-mentioned elements in addition to extra vitamins if these are indicated.

DIETS FOR CHILDREN

► **A Sample Day's Meals for a 4-Year-Old**

BREAKFAST

Orange.

Oatmeal (½ cup) with milk (⅛ cup).

Whole-wheat toast (2 thin slices) with butter or fortified margarine (2 teaspoonfuls).
Milk (½ pint).

DINNER

Ground beef ball (1 small) or boneless fish.
Baked potato (1 small) with butter or fortified margarine (1 teaspoonful).
Green beans (¼ cup) with butter or fortified margarine (½ teaspoonful).
Custard (⅓ cup).
Milk (½ pint).

SUPPER

Poached egg.
Carrot strips (3 pieces).
Enriched bread (1 slice) with butter or fortified margarine (1 teaspoonful).
Applesauce (½ cup) with milk (2 tablespoonfuls).
Milk (½ pint).

▶ A Sample Day's Meals for a 10-Year-Old

BREAKFAST

Tomato juice (¾ cup).
Hot whole-wheat cereal (⅔ cup) with milk (½ cup).
Toast (2 slices) with butter or fortified margarine (2 teaspoonfuls).
Milk (½ pint).

LUNCH

(If served at school or at home)
Creamed eggs (¾ cup).
Green beans (½ cup) with butter or fortified margarine (1 teaspoonful).
Oatmeal muffins (2) with butter or fortified margarine (2 teaspoonfuls).
Milk (½ pint).

(If brought from home)
Sandwich—peanut butter and raw carrot on buttered whole-grain or enriched bread.
Sandwich—chopped dried fruit on buttered whole-grain or enriched bread.

Supplemented at school by—
  Orange.
  Milk soup (1 cup) or cocoa (1 cup).

DINNER
  Meat loaf (1 serving).
  Scalloped potatoes (⅔ cup).
  Cole slaw with red and green peppers (½ cup).
  Whole-wheat bread or enriched bread (2 slices) with butter
    or fortified margarine (2 teaspoonfuls).
  Applesauce (½ cup).
  Molasses cookies (2 thin).
  Milk (½ pint).

Reprinted from *Nutrition and Healthy Growth,* Children's Bureau publication, U.S. Department of Health, Education, and Welfare.

DIETS, VITAMINS AND ESSENTIAL MINERALS   Vitamins and minerals are essential chemicals in the diet, and are found in foods. They are crucial in the formation of the structure of muscles, bones, tissues and various organs of the body. Vitamin and mineral deficiencies cause specific diseases. A well-balanced diet containing all the various vitamins and minerals is the best protection against these diseases. In childhood, supplementary vitamins and minerals are taken as added protection against deficiencies. Unless there is a poor dietary intake, poor absorption due to gastroenteritis, vomiting, celiac syndrome, or increased excretion of vitamins, a normal well-balanced diet will provide adequate nutrients for good nutrition and growth.

VITAMIN A. Deficiencies of vitamin A may cause, among other symptoms, dryness and scaliness of the skin, and small, dry spots on the conjunctiva. Vitamin A poisoning or hypervitaminosis is a condition caused by a history of prolonged and excessive dosage of vitamin A. The treatment for vitamin A poisoning is to stop the administration of vitamin A. Sources of vitamin are milk, beef, liver, egg yolk and various fish oils.

VITAMIN B₁ (THIAMINE CHLORIDE). Severe deficiency of this vitamin causes beriberi, which may affect the heart and peripheral nerves. Sources of vitamin B_1 are milk, liver, pork, eggs, vegetables, wheat bran, soybeans, and fruits.

VITAMIN B₂ (RIBOFLAVIN). Riboflavin deficiency may produce various eye symptoms alone or in combination, such as burning, itching, difficulty in looking at light (photophobia), cracks at the corner of the mouth, ulcers and fissures at the corners and inside the mucous membranes of the mouth, greasy scales on reddish skin, particularly around the nose, or a magenta-colored, smooth, painful tongue. Sources of riboflavin are milk, liver, pork, eggs, vegetables, cereals and fruit.

VITAMIN C (ASCORBIC ACID). Deficiency in vitamin C causes scurvy. This is a disease of increased capillary fragility in which there are hemorrhages under the lining of the bone (subperiosteal). Good sources of vitamin C are citrus fruit and tomatoes.

VITAMIN D (ANTIRACHITIC VITAMIN). Early signs of vitamin D deficiency occur in the skull, with softening and thinning of the bone, so that when it is pressed in, it cracks like a ping pong ball. Later signs of rickets show bulging of the frontal (forehead) bones, pigeon breast, and grooves in the rib insertions of the diaphragm. The legs are usually bowed, and walking is usually difficult. Vitamin D is found in fish, fish-liver oils, sunlight, and activated steroids.

VITAMIN K. A lack of this important vitamin may cause a bleeding disorder in the newborn child. Administration of synthetic vitamin K to the mother before delivery, and later to the newborn infant, will prevent this condition. Vitamin K is found in many foods and especially in cabbage, cauliflower, liver, pork, soybeans, spinach, and alfalfa.

NIACIN (NICOTINIC ACID). This is the anti-pellagra factor. Symptoms of niacin deficiency may be found singly or in combinations, pellagra itself being characterized by dermatitis, diarrhea, and dementia. Poor power of concentration, mental confusion, irritability and depression may occur. Sources of niacin in diet are liver, meat, whole milk, and wheat.

BIOTIN. Deficiency of biotin in humans is rare but if present will cause skin lesions, lassitude, and muscle pain. Good sources of biotin are beef liver, roasted peanuts, chocolate, and eggs.

FOLIC ACID. Deficiency may result in megaloblastic erythropoesis. Good sources of folic acid are meat and chicken livers, wheat bran, asparagus and dry lima beans.

PANTOTHENIC ACID. Because almost any daily diet contains foods with a pantothenic acid content, deficiency signs in humans are not fully identified, but evidence exists that dizziness, constipation, and numbness of hands and feet are among some of the symptoms produced by pantothenic acid deficiency. Almost all foods are sources of pantothenic acid, but especially beef and pork liver, wheat germ, lamb kidney, and broccoli.

VITAMIN B_6 (PYRIDOXINE). Deficiency, although rare, could produce seborrheic dermatitis in the area of the eyes and mouth. Sources of vitamin B_6 are blackstrap molasses, soybeans, wheat bran, and whole rice.

VITAMIN B_{12}. Deficiency of vitamin B_{12} may result in some form of anemia. Good sources of vitamin B_{12} are meat livers, meat kidneys, and fish.

MINERALS. Deficiency or absence in the diet of the essential minerals may cause metabolic disruptions with associated diseases. The essential minerals (some sources of each mineral are given in the parentheses) are calcium (milk), phosphorus (almonds, whole wheat grain), magnesium (cocoa, peanuts, whole wheat flour), sodium (salt), potassium (eggs, meats, skim milk, soybean flours), manganese (oatmeal, whole wheat flour), iron (beef, lamb, and hog liver, soybean flours, yeast), copper (liver, oysters), cobalt (cabbage, spinach, lettuce), iodine (iodized salt), sulfur (eggs, chicken, salmon), zinc (herrings, wheat bran, yeast), and flourine (mackerel, salmon, sardines).

DILATATION AND CURETTAGE (D&C)   This is a surgical procedure in which part or most of the lining of the uterus is removed. It is sometimes referred to by the layman as a "scraping." The procedure is done by the vaginal route. In essence it consists of dilating the os, *i.e.,* the opening of the uterus. Next the curette—a long rod with a shallow cuplike head—is introduced into the uterine cavity and portions of the lining removed.

A D&C is an important and useful diagnostic procedure, since the tissue removed can be examined for abnormalities. Thus, in the presence of abnormal or frequent uterine bleeding, a D&C may be necessary to determine which of many possible conditions may be present. By examining tissue samples it may be possible to determine the existence of chronic hormonal stimulation, polyp formation, cancer, chronic inflammation, or the presence of benign tumors known as fibroids. Some cases of continued bleeding after childbirth are due to retention within the uterus of parts of the placenta. It may be necessary to remove these by a curettage.

In addition to its value in diagnosis, a D&C may also cure certain abnormal conditions of the lining. A thorough scraping will remove all the abnormal tissue and leave the uterus in a state somewhat similar to that at the end of menstruation. A more normal cycle of growth and development in the lining may then follow. A D&C performed on a pregnant woman is known as an abortion. Where menstrual cycles have been irregular and the possibility of pregnancy exists, many hospitals may require a pregnancy test before permitting a D&C. This is done to rule out the possibility of unwittingly tampering with an early pregnancy.

The course of events after the D&C somewhat resembles those of a menstrual period. Several days of bleeding, necessitating the wearing of a napkin, generally follow. Bleeding that is unusually heavy or profuse, or fever and discharge, should be reported to the doctor. The procedure itself is generally done in a hospital setting. An injection to prevent pain or some brief form of general anesthesia is generally required. In the usual course of events the patient will be discharged within a day or so.

DIPHTHERIA   *Cause.* Bacterial, *Corynebacterium diphtheriae.*

Incubation period. 2 to 7 days.

Symptoms. This disease is spread by contact with cases or carriers. The symptoms are caused by a membrane which forms on the tonsils, pharynx, and lining of the throat. This narrows breathing capacity and also produces a toxin (poison) which is absorbed by the blood and causes the most severe symptoms of this disease. In order to neutralize this poison, diphtheria antitoxin has to be used early in the disease. Otherwise the antitoxin will have no effect. The diphtheria toxin has a special attraction for cardiac (heart), renal (kidney), and nervous tissues.

Diphtheria in the throat area is characterized first by swelling of the tonsils and glands of the neck, with pus spots and a yellowish white membrane covering the tonsils. Fever, rapid heart rate, malaise, and weakness occur. Classical symptoms of croup with noisy, obstructed breathing, brassy cough, hoarseness, and "pulling" (retractions) of the chest follow. This is caused by obstruction to the air passages. If this obstruction is not relieved, death may result from heart failure, exhaustion, or choking.

Diphtheria is rare during the first six months of life, as passive immunity is obtained by the newborn child from antibodies of the mother (if the mother is immune). If the mother is susceptible to diphtheria, so is the child. Diphtheria occurs in epidemics throughout the world and is more frequent in the winter. The sickness and death rate from diphtheria has declined rapidly in the United States since 1920, when active immunization became widely established. Not everyone who recovers from diphtheria develops immunity, and secondary attacks have been known to occur. The Schick test was developed to test whether a person is susceptible to diphtheria. It is not in general use today because immunization is so widespread.

Complications. These may include paralysis as a result of peripheral neuritis. Selective paralysis of eye muscles, palate, and other areas of the body may occur.

Treatment. Cases of diphtheria should be hospitalized. Antitoxin, antibiotics, and oxygen may be required. In severe cases, tracheotomy (an operation to open the windpipe) may be necessary. This operation makes an artificial airway into the trachea below the area blocked by the membrane in the throat.

Prevention. Immunization with diphtheria toxoid should be started within the first year of life, followed by booster doses every two to three years. This may be administered in the form of triple toxoid or individual diphtheria toxoid. Children who have been exposed to diphtheria should be Schick-tested, and those with positive Schick tests should receive passive immunization.

DIVERTICULITIS   A diverticulum (plural, diverticula) is an outpouching of an organ, generally with an internal lining similar to that of the organ itself. Common locations for diverticula are in the urinary bladder and in any portion of the digestive tract including the esophagus, stomach, and small and large intestine.

By far the most common location is the large intestine. Indeed, diverticula of the colon are found in such a large number of middle-aged individuals that they are not considered particularly unusual. They are generally multiple and more common in the descending colon, which is on the left side of the abdomen, but do occur at other points. On an X-ray of the large intestine they generally appear as tiny outgrowths on slim stalks. Even the wider ones are generally considerably smaller than a small grape. Ordinarily their presence arouses no concern. In a few individuals, and for reasons that are not always clear, diverticula may become inflamed, producing the condition known as diverticulitis. This occurs perhaps more commonly in the lower left fourth of the abdomen, so that diverticulitis is sometimes referred to as "left-sided appendicitis." There may be crampy abdominal pain, tenderness in the affected region, and some degree of fever.

Treatment. Diverticulitis is most often treated conservatively by putting the digestive tract to rest, giving feedings intravenously, by use of antibiotics, and similar measures. It is seldom necessary to operate. Rarely, local abscess-formation or some degree of intestinal obstruction may necessitate surgery. However, the chances are thousands to one against surgery becoming necessary. Another (equally rare) complication of diverticulitis is bleeding; a history of passing blood with the bowel movement may lead the doctor to consider diverticulitis as a possible cause. Generally no special diet or alteration in the way of life is made necessary by the presence of diverticula. It is generally advised that constipation be avoided, perhaps by taking a stool softener or doses of mineral oil.

▶ **Meckel's Diverticulum** Meckel's diverticulum is a rather small protrusion from the small intestine near the ileocecal valve. It may remain quiet as an unnecessary remnant, or it may produce symptoms. It may produce the same symptoms as an acutely inflamed appendix, or give the signs and symptoms of acute intestinal obstruction. It may bleed, producing the picture of a bleeding ulcer. It is usually only diagnosed during surgery, when it can be observed and confirmed.

DIZZINESS, MOTION SICKNESS Dizziness is also known as motion sickness and technically as vertigo. True vertigo arises from a disturbance of the semicircular canals located in the inner ear or of the nerve pathways running from it to the brain centers. The canals are filled with a fluid which, if set into sudden or violent motion, may produce sensations of giddiness and nausea. When vertigo is marked, the patient will complain that everything seems to be reeling, his gait may stagger, and his nausea may increase and lead to vomiting. He may be unable to remain upright and even when lying down may complain of dizziness which is increased by every motion of the head.

Motion sickness refers to this disturbance when it is produced as a result of the movement of the body through space, and is commonly encountered on shipboard—sea-sickness—and occasionally in autos—car sickness. Generally children are more susceptible to car sickness than adults.

In certain viral respiratory illnesses, the semicircular canals may be involved and extreme dizziness may result. This condition, sometimes referred to as labyrinthitis, may also be encountered after the use of certain drugs, such as the barbiturates, or large doses of alcohol. A severe form of labyrinthitis which comes in episodes, particularly in middle age and later, is known as Meniere's syndrome. The person may be suddenly seized with severe dizziness, nausea, and vomiting and may be completely incapacitated.

Various other sensations in the head are sometimes incorrectly described as dizziness. These include certain forms of lightheadedness to which individuals with low or very high blood pressures may be subject, and the somewhat similar sensations complained of when sleep has been inadequate or as a result of a "hangover" from either alcohol or sleeping pills. Elderly persons with some evidence of hardening of the arteries may have bouts of unsteadiness described as "dizziness."

Treatment. For motion sickness, Meniere's syndrome, and allied disorders there are several drugs useful in prevention or treatment. They should not be taken, however, without the advice of a physician.

128

DOUCHE   A douche is the introduction into the vagina of a watery solution of a medication or drug. It is no longer considered necessary or even desirable for a woman to douche unless some special indication for it is present. It would be well to discuss the advisability of douching with the doctor; some physicians advise against it at any time during pregnancy, except in very special circumstances.

Douches are most often advised in the following situations: (1) Vaginitis, or vaginal infections by certain organisms. Here the douche is generally medicated. Sometimes a simple vinegar douche, made by adding three tablespoons of white vinegar to two quarts of warm water, may be prescribed. Or various medicines or specially prepared powders may be advised. (2) Excessive secretions, such as may necessitate the wearing of a sanitary napkin. Here, a cleansing douche is sometimes prescribed. (3) Douches are sometimes used as a birth-control measure. Such douching, however, is not reliable: whatever advantage is gained by it calls for its immediate use after intercourse.

Douching requires a bag with rubber tubing connected to a hard rubber or plastic nozzle. A cutoff clamp on the rubber tubing will also prove useful. Douching is most conveniently carried out in a bathtub. The douche bag should be no higher than two feet above the level of the hips. After making up the solution in the bag, preferably at about body temperature, the nozzle is inserted approximately two or three inches into the vagina. No attempt should be made to bring the lips of the vagina around the tubing, as free escape of the fluid is necessary.

A convenient position for douching is to recline in the tub with the knees partially drawn up. The douche fluid is allowed to circulate freely into and out of the vagina. It is seldom necessary to douche more than several times a week and often less. For certain kinds of stubborn vaginal infection, daily douching may be prescribed by the doctor.

DRUGS AND REMEDIES

▶ **Antibiotics**   An antibiotic is a substance secreted by one organism which will kill other organisms—specifically bacteria and fungi. The first and best-known of the antibiotics is penicillin. Its successors include streptomycin, tetracycline, and terramycin. Less well known are mycostatin, griseofulvin, kanamycin, and others which have limited but useful special application. Recently, chemically modified forms of the naturally occurring penicillin have appeared; these have useful new properties, including the ability to attack certain penicillin-resistant organisms.

The sulfonamide drugs preceded the antibiotics, then for a long time were displaced by them. They are synthetic chemicals which come out of the chemists' test tube and not out of a fermentation vat. Between the antibiotics and the sulfa drugs, today's doctor has a wide choice of infection-fighting agents. These drugs can be used against an almost endless list of infections, ranging from pimples and boils to pneumonia and meningitis. Constant advances are made in the antibiotic field. Thus at one time streptomycin was extensively used in the treatment of tuberculosis but has now been largely supplanted by a very simple chemical related to one of the vitamin B group—isonicotinic hydrazide (INH). Some antibiotics should be used only when all other measures fail; thus, although griseofulvin is effective when taken by mouth for the treatment of athlete's foot and similar fungus infections, one would certainly try local measures first.

The most important limiting factor in the treatment of infections is the absence of agents that will kill off viruses. For instance, there is no presently available drug that can be used in the treatment of acute poliomyelitis, measles, influenza, the common cold, and other virus-produced illnesses. The first step the doctor must take is to decide the nature of an infection; only then can an antibiotic drug be correctly prescribed.

Sometimes a resistant organism is encountered which does not respond to the usual antibiotic. The usual countermeasure is either to increase the dose or switch to another antibiotic. There are also certain drawbacks to be kept in mind: at least 5 per cent of the population will develop an allergy to penicillin. This may be manifested by hives, joint pains, fever, and occasionally by a collapse following a penicillin injection. Tetracycline may occasionally produce somewhat similar reactions, and in addition may encourage an overgrowth of certain organisms usually kept in check. This may result in diarrhea or in vaginal itching. With pregnant women it is now generally considered a good rule to take drugs only for good reason and under a doctor's direction.

▶ **Anticoagulants** These form an important group of drugs which diminish the clotting power of the blood. They can prevent the extension of a clot that has already formed, or can be used prophylactically to prevent clots. Heparin was the first drug with anticoagulant properties to be used. It has to be given by injection and produces a prompt drop in the co-agulability of the blood. Because of its expense and the necessity for injection, another group of drugs without these disadvantages has been developed (dicumarol, coumadin, and others). With these it is possible to maintain long-term treatment, and some patients have been on anticoagulant drugs for years.

The correct dose of the drug to be taken is arrived at by frequent testing of blood samples. It is impossible to predict in advance how much will be needed. Sometimes the dose has to be changed because of fluctuations in blood clotting capacity. In overdose there may be noted easy bruising, so that black-and-blue marks appear in the skin with slight bumps or even without apparent injuries. Bleeding in the urinary tract with reddish urine, and occasionally into the digestive tract with a reddish-to-blackish stool, may also occur from overdosage. This is easily corrected by giving the appropriate antidote, vitamin K. The great majority of patients do very well on anticoagulants. Some can be allowed to go for relatively long periods of time between routine checks. Hence the need for testing may diminish from almost daily down to weekly and even monthly.

Clotting (thrombosis) in a large vein is one common condition for which anticoagulants may be prescribed. Thrombosis is more likely to occur in patients who are compelled to stay in bed for days or weeks, as in the treatment of a heart attack. Some, though not all, doctors may consider it worthwhile to give such a patient an anticoagulant drug. The drugs have also been used, though again there are differences of opinion here, for the long-term treatment of patients who have had a heart attack. It is felt that there may be less risk of a second attack if the clotting power of the blood is diminished. Recent studies suggest that this particular effect diminishes considerably after the first year.

In certain elderly individuals, impaired circulation to the brain results in transient bouts of visual difficulties, weakness, and dizziness; anticoagulants seem to be useful in cutting down and even eliminating such episodes. However, if high blood pressure is present, it is generally considered less safe to use the anticoagulants. Since the anticoagulants are relatively recent drugs on the medical scene, precise opinions as to their range of usage are still being formed.

▶ **Barbiturates** The important chemical compound, barbituric acid, was synthesized at the turn of the century; it and its derivatives are widely used in medical practice. They have sedative and sleep-producing properties and, although much maligned and abused, are important and useful drugs. Collectively, these compounds are known as the barbiturates. Perhaps the best known is phenobarbital, widely employed as a sedative. In moderate doses it allays anxiety and is hence used to assuage feelings of tension, restlessness, and for sleep difficulties. It may produce some dulling, with feelings of drowsiness. It is also useful in psychosomatic disturbances—that is, in such disorders as "nervous headaches," "nervous stomach," spastic colitis—and has some value in the treatment of nausea. Hence many of the compounds used for the treatment of disorders of the digestive tract incorporate phenobarbital as one of the ingredients. It is also used to diminish overstimulation produced by such drugs as ephedrine, a medication used in the treatment of asthma and other conditions. In some patients use of phenobarbital may produce a rash.

The other widespread application of the barbiturates is in the treatment of insomnia and other sleep disorders. A dose of one of these compounds taken at bedtime will generally induce sleep, often for five or more hours. Depending on dosage and individual response, one may awake feeling refreshed or somewhat sleepy and heavy-headed. Some tolerance generally develops to sleeping pills after they have been taken for a time. In ordinary dosages, however, there is no danger of addiction or habit formation. Those who have to take sleeping pills night after night do not do so because of addiction, but rather because the reasons for insomnia (whatever they may be) are often constant and well-established ones. Hence, whatever produces the need for sleeping pills in the beginning will again become apparent if the sleeping pills are omitted.

▶ **Diuretics**   Diuretics are substances which increase the production of urine. The caffeine found in coffee and tea and the theobromine found in cocoa are examples of natural diuretic substances. Certain a c i d i f y i n g salts, of which ammonium chloride is an example, will also increase urine production. Much more potent diuretics than these are now available. A single dose may lead to a 3 to 5-pint increase in urine production within the following twenty-four hours. This in turn would mean a 3 to 5-pound loss of body weight, since a pint of fluid weighs a pound.

The first potent group of diuretics were known as the mercurial diuretics, since their active ingredient was an organic compound of mercury. Mercurial diuretics are generally given by injection and induce a very prompt and often extensive urinary increase. In recent years some potent drugs which are effective by mouth have been synthesized. They are sometimes collectively referred to as the chlorothiazide group of drugs. One or two of these pills may produce a diuresis equivalent to that following a mercurial drug. In addition to promoting the excretion of sodium chloride, which is common salt, these pills also increase the excretion of potassium from the body. To compensate for this the pills may be combined with potassium salts. Otherwise their frequent or long-continued use may lead to states of serious potassium depletion, manifested by muscular weakness.

Diuretics are invaluable drugs in all fields of medicine. With them it is possible to get rid of fluid accumulations which otherwise may be annoying, troublesome, or even massive. Diuretics may be used by women with troublesome fluid accumulations during the last part of their menstrual cycles. Also during pregnancy, when fluid accumulation is marked or the blood pressure is rising too high, the doctor may prescribe diuretics. A clot in a large vein of the lower extremity may result in troublesome chronic leg swelling. This too may be controlled, at least partially, by the diuretics.

A second most important application of these drugs is in the treatment of high blood pressure. For reasons that are not entirely clear, promoting the excretion of salt and water from the body tends to lower blood pressure. Hence these drugs are one of the basic approaches in the drug treatment of hypertension. On the whole they produce relatively few unpleasant effects. Sometimes, when the rate of urine production is quite brisk, muscular cramps due to rapid loss of salts may be noted. This may be an indication for decreasing the dose somewhat. Diuretic drugs, however, should not be taken for trivial reasons, nor without some form of medical supervision.

▶ **Laxatives** Laxatives are agents which promote the evacuation of the large intestine. The old distinction drawn between laxatives, cathartics, and purgatives is not a practical one. Originally the laxatives were regarded as the least active and the purgatives as the most active evacuants. The distinction is in part due to dosage; a small dose of a specific medicine will have a mild laxative effect, but increasing it may produce a great number of watery stools—a purgative action. There are many stimulants that move the bowel, and their mechanisms of action are different. Thus castor oil stimulates the muscle of the small intestine as well as the large one, and produces copious watery movements. In addition, it stimulates the muscle of the uterus and hence should not be used during pregnancy. Other laxatives have a bulk or mechanical effect.

One classification based upon action is the following:

1. *Saline cathartics.* These draw fluid out into the intestinal canal because of their salt concentration, and so will produce one or more bowel movements that are more watery than usual. Saline cathartics include Epsom salts (magnesium sulphate), phospho-soda (sodium phosphate), citrate of magnesia (magnesium citrate solution), and Seidlitz powders (potassium and sodium tartrate).

2. *Bulk-lubricant group.* These increase the bulk of the intestinal contents, hence stimulate the bowel to evacuation and may have a lubricating effect. Mineral oil is a common example of this. Other bulk agents include bran, psyllium or its extracts, and agar.

3. *Stool-softeners.* These are wetting agents which keep the stool moist and therefore bulkier. They are usually taken daily, are well tolerated, and are used in all age groups including babies. With them the small, hard, or pellety stool of chronic constipation becomes larger, bulkier, and moister.

4. *Irritant cathartics.* These include many plant extracts and fruits such as prunes used for centuries in the treatment of constipation.

5. *Suppositories.* These are sometimes a convenient way of emptying the rectum promptly.

▶ **Steroid Drugs** The two hormones of the ovary, a group of adrenal hormones, and the male hormone all bear considerable resemblance to each other.

These hormones are collectively spoken of as the "steroid hormones."

▶ **Sulfonamide (Sulfa) Drugs** This is a group of germ-killing drugs created synthetically and first introduced in the early 1930's. The first one, sulfanilamide, is now of historical importance only and has been succeeded by a number of derivatives with varying properties. For a time the sulfonamide drugs were pushed aside by the new antibiotics, but they are now returning to their rightful place and have widespread usage. In some cases they are good alternatives to the antibiotics. Thus, in children who have had rheumatic fever, a daily dose of penicillin or a sulfonamide drug should be taken to prevent recurrences. If the child is sensitive to penicillin, he will have no choice except to take the sulfa drug. For many urinary tract infections, infections of the sinuses, sore throats, etc., the choice of whether it is to be a sulfa drug or an antibiotic may be in part a matter of personal preference on the part of the physician. He will be guided especially by any knowledge of past difficulties with the drugs that the patient may have experienced: reactions such as nausea, vaginal itching, or drug eruptions. In meningitis and certain other infections the sulfa drugs may be the preferred ones.

Most of the sulfa drugs have to be taken at frequent intervals, perhaps every four to six hours, since they tend to be rapidly excreted through the urine; it is sometimes advised that extra water be drunk to prevent any crystallization of the drug in the urine. Recently, longer-acting and more slowly excreted derivatives have been created which need be taken only once every twelve hours.

There is also a group of poorly absorbed sulfonamide drugs which can be taken by mouth in large quantities. These are particularly effective in infections of the intestinal tract. Because of poor absorption from the intestine, large amounts can be given and high concentrations achieved. This property is useful in certain dysenteries and in preparing the intestine for certain operative procedures; these drugs are sometimes referred to as the intestinal sulfonamides. In certain severe infections, a sulfonamide drug can be injected directly into the vein for high concentrations in the bloodstream.

▶ **Tranquilizers** A tranquilizer is a drug which will diminish nervous tension and its manifestations. A perfect tranquilizer would diminish anxiety without impairing the ability to think. In practice, depending in part on the drug and the person taking it, some slowing up or sedative effect is likely to be noted. There is, therefore, only a difference of degree between some of the new tranquilizers and some of the older sedative drugs, such as phenobarbital. This difference may be of some value, since there may be less sleepiness with a tranquilizer. Hence, for the woman who has difficulty falling asleep, a tranquilizer might be preferred if she wants to get up during the night to give the baby a formula; after the usual dose of a barbiturate a woman might find herself too sleepy or dizzy to function well. A distinction is sometimes drawn between minor tranquilizers—such as meprobamate (Miltown®, Equanil®), which is used for minor symptoms of anxiety like nervous headache, jitteriness, difficulty in falling asleep, etc.—and major tranquilizers which can be used in severe mental disturbances, such as states of great agitation and overactivity or various psychotic disorders.

The first major tranquilizer—and still one of the most widely employed—is thorazine. Various drugs, some more or less closely related to thorazine, have appeared in the last ten years and have greatly improved treatment of mental disorders. In full dosage, such as may be given only in a hospital setting, a major tranquilizer may greatly suppress delusions, hallucinations, and hyperactivity in an agitated psychotic. Through their use, long periods of institutionalization have been so drastically cut that the major tranquilizers are said to have introduced a new era in the treatment of mental disorders. Small doses of tranquilizers may be effective against nausea.

EAR CONDITIONS

▶ **Hearing Disability** There may be organic causes for hearing defects, such as ear malformations, trauma, infections and diseases of the nose, throat, and ear. Other defects due to hereditary or birth injuries may cause a delay in hearing. This, of course, will cause delay in speech development.

It is difficult to discover a hearing defect in a very young infant. However, most parents will be able to tell whether the child wakes on hearing a loud noise, or responds to music or the sound of a voice. As a child approaches school age, accurate audiometric evaluation (hearing tests) is possible. It is extremely necessary to treat all ear infections in children until they are cleared, otherwise many such infections may result in impaired hearing.

Treatment of hearing defects includes speech therapy, lip reading, acoustic training, hearing aids, and sometimes schooling in a special school for the hard-of-hearing.

▶ **Otitis (Ear Infection)**   The ear is divided into the external, middle, and internal (inner) ear. These units conduct sound and maintain equilibrium. Acute otitis media is a term describing inflammation of the lining membrane of the middle ear. It is usually a result of an infection carried from the throat or tonsil area through the eustachian tube. In children, the most outstanding symptom is ear pain which results from pressure of fluid behind the drum, or from inflammation of the drum. Hearing may be impaired, and sometimes noises and ringing may be heard.

In small infants who have no demonstrable sign of illness, fretting, crying, screaming with pain, head-banging, or handling of the ear may indicate an ear infection. It can only be diagnosed by looking into the ear with an otoscope.

Ear infections should be treated with antibiotics. If they are not treated early, pus accumulates behind the eardrum, the drum may rupture, and chronic draining ear may develop. This will predispose to the development of mastoiditis and possibly meningitis. Hearing loss and deafness may also develop.

▶ **Acute Mastoiditis**   Acute mastoiditis usually occurs as a complication of middle ear infections. Since the advent of antibiotics, which usually cure most middle ear infections, it has become a rare condition.

The signs of this condition are: persistent fever, pain in the ear and behind the ear, hearing loss, and general toxicity. There is tenderness over the mastoid area (the bone just behind the ear) and X-ray will show destruction of the mastoid cells. If pus discharges from the ear and remains untreated, mastoiditis is very likely to develop. The treatment is usually surgery plus antibiotics.

EYES—CROSS-EYES OR SQUINT (STRABISMUS)

Squint is caused by abnormalities in the nerves or the ocular muscles. The person fixes one eye on an object while the other eye turns so that the image does not fall on the center portion of the eye. This condition may involve one or both eyes.

Paralytic squint is due to either partial or complete paralysis of one or more of the eye muscles. This may cause a turning of the eye to one side, double vision, or restriction of motion.

Concomitant squint is a muscle imbalance which involves both eyes equally. It does not involve paralysis or loss of function of one single muscle. These squints may be intermittent or alternating, converging or diverging and/or vertical. In children this condition is usually caused by an imbalance between the ciliary muscle and the internal recti muscles.

Treatment. Surgical treatment is usually necessary if the squint has been present since birth. Early surgery, between the ages of two and three years, produces a better result and prevents more complications. Since the brain and cerebral structures are involved in correct eye functioning, a delay in surgery may lead to loss of vision in one of the eyes.

Medical treatment alone is usually only successful in infants who have developed cross-eyes after the age of eighteen or twenty-four months. It is possible to test eyes of infants and young children to determine whether they require glasses. Sometimes glasses will convert squinting eyes to normal. However, training and special eye exercises may often be necessary in addition to glasses.

EYES, INFLAMMATION OF

▶ **Conjunctivitis** Conjunctivitis is an inflammation of the conjunctiva, the lining of the eye. In health the conjunctiva appears pale and glistening; it has relatively few visible blood vessels traversing it. As a result of the inflammation it turns quite red (hence the term "pink eye"), and whitish or yellowish secretion may accumulate. Sometimes, particularly after a night's sleep, the accumulated secretion may fuse the eyelashes together to such an extent that opening the eye is difficult or temporarily impossible. Washing this dried exudate away will generally relieve this condition. Conjunctivitis can result from the irritation of chemicals, smoke, or dusts, and is occasionally allergic in origin. Most cases, however, are due to inflammations set up by various bacteria. Thus, epidemics of conjunctivitis have been reported due to a germ known as the Koch-Weeks bacillus. More common organisms such as the staphylococcus and the streptococcus are also to be found in isolated cases of conjunctivitis. In many instances conjunctivitis occurs in both eyes, or if it appears in one eye first it will not infrequently spread to the other.

Treatment. Mild cases due to smoke, dusts, and mechanical irritants will subside by themselves. Even mild cases due to bacterial inflammation may not require special treatment, since the bodily defenses can generally handle them. It is possible to get a very high local concentration of a sulfa drug or an antibiotic into the area of conjunctivitis, however. A drop or two from an eyedropper will do this, and as a rule conjunctivitis will respond quite promptly to instillations of such drugs.

As a precaution against the possibility of the newborn baby developing conjunctivitis from an unsuspected gonorrheal infection in the mother, many states require that silver nitrate drops be placed in the eyes immediately after birth. This routine has virtually eliminated gonorrheal conjunctivitis in the newborn. Infants may acquire other forms of conjunctivitis, however, including some due to viruses. Generally speaking, none of these is serious, and response to treatment is generally prompt and satisfactory.

▶ **Sty** This is an inflammation and infection of the eyelid. A hair follicle may become red, enlarged, and cause an accumulation of pus. The eyelid becomes red and painful; tears and a pus discharge may occur.

Treatment. Warm boric acid eyewashes, or compresses, in addition to antibiotics by mouth and by injections will usually suffice.

EYES—VISUAL DIFFICULTIES Most visual difficulties can be understood only if one has some basic knowledge of the structures within the eye. The eye can be compared to the camera; it has a clear portion admitting light (the cornea), a variable lens opening (the pupil, controlled by the iris), and beyond this a lens whose thickness can be modified and which throws the image onto the back part of the eye (the retina). Difficulties in focusing the image correctly are called refractive errors. Compensating lenses can partially or wholly correct such errors, and these are the lenses we wear as eyeglasses.

Common refractive errors include:

1. *Myopia.* In this condition the eyeball is relatively long so that the image transmitted through the lens focuses in front of the retina. It is corrected by a concave lens (thinner in the middle than at the sides). Myopia runs in some families and has a hereditary aspect.

2. *Hypermetropia.* This condition is known as farsightedness. Here the reverse of myopia exists, the eyeball being somewhat shorter than it should be. The visual difficulty is most marked with images that are close up, not with objects that are at a distance. A lens which is convex, the opposite of the one used for nearsightedness, will be prescribed for this condition.

3. *Presbyopia.* There is a loss of elasticity in the lens of the eye as we grow older. Because of this some of its power to focus on nearby objects is lost past the age of forty to fifty. Fine print cannot be read at the usual distance, though for a time it may be readable when held out at arm's length. A lens similar to that used for farsightedness will help—"reading glasses."

4. *Astigmatism.* Slight distortions in the cornea, the transparent window-like opening at the front of the eye, will produce blurring in some parts of the transmitted image. It may be associated with other difficulties but may also exist alone.

Various conditions, such as fatigue or some illnesses, may affect the refractive behavior of the eye. Some people do not focus as well when they are very tired or when they first get up in the morning. Diabetes, by temporarily altering the various fluids within the eyeball, may lead to a refractive error which is correctable when the diabetes is brought under control. In addition, diabetes tends to increase the rate at which cataracts (opacifications) form within the lens. Some of the antispasmodic drugs may cut down on the ability to focus; this is also temporary and reversible.

▶ **Blindness** The most extreme visual difficulty is, of course, blindness. Recognition of blindness in a young infant may be difficult within the first few months. After that, it can be rec-

140

ognized by a failure to respond to normal stimulation by the parent. The child does not smile appropriately or follow objects with his eyes and appears to stare vacantly.

Blind children present special problems in learning and development. Blindness also creates emotional problems for the parents, family, and friends. Blind children require specialized schools which teach them to develop a sense of independence and self-sufficiency. At such schools they are taught touch systems (the Braille alphabet) of reading and special methods of getting around in the street. The parents as well as the children must learn how to handle the problem of the visually handicapped. Given proper training, blind children can grow up into useful, productive adults.

FAINTING   A fainting episode is associated with a marked drop in blood pressure which results in a temporary decline in the circulation to the brain. Hot and crowded surroundings, a painful injection, a sudden unpleasant sight or upsetting news are among the common causes. There may be some warning signals, such as pallor, perspiration, complaints of dizziness, or "spots before the eyes." If the victim is quickly stretched out or if the head is lowered at once, fainting may be avoided. Otherwise unconsciousness may ensue, sometimes in association with brief muscular twitching.

Cold applications, chafing of the hands and forearms, and allowing the person to inhale aromatic spirits of ammonia are old, well-established measures. The losses of consciousness just described are sometimes called simple faints. They are to be differentiated from fainting due to such causes as bleeding, internal hemorrhage, overdoses of insulin, and other episodes which will require medical attention.

FALLS AND FRACTURES   It is not always possible to tell whether a fall has resulted in a bruise, a sprain, or a serious fracture—a break in the bone. A fracture may be looked for when a person has fallen from a considerable height or has suffered severe or multiple impacts, as in falling down stairs or in auto accidents. However, in the elderly fractures may occur with relatively little impact because of brittleness of the bones in old age. A fracture may also be suspected if there is an obvious deformity, a shortening of an extremity, or if crepitus (a grating sound) is produced on gentle touching of the injured part. *If there is any possibility of a fracture involving the backbone, no attempts should be made to move the person or to help him to his feet,* as occasionally serious damage to the spinal cord may occur.

For other fractures, immobilization by splints is necessary before any movement is attempted. The splints can be sticks of wood, boughs, broom handles, umbrellas, or anything else which can be satisfactorily applied to the limb. The splint is placed so as to run to the joint above and the joint below the site of the fracture and so that it can be secured in place with handkerchiefs, twine, or any other binding available.

Where only bruises and sprains have resulted from the injury, the best first-aid measure is application of cold. Thus, compresses wrung out of icewater or an icebag may be applied to the area. Cold can be maintained continuously (or intermittently, if uncomfortable) for hours; it results in diminishing pain, swelling, and bleeding. Generally, starting in about twenty-four hours, local heat can be used. This may be in the form of a heating pad, hot wet compresses, or a heat lamp. Heat treatments may be given for as long as a half hour and can be repeated several times a day. An X-ray of the region may be necessary to rule out fracture. Aspirin and other pain-killing medications are frequently necessary.

FEVER   Even an everyday event like fever still defies complete explanation. Most often, in the presence of infection, the temperature-regulating center in the mid-brain, which functions like a thermostat, allows the "setting" to go somewhat higher. It is thought that higher body temperatures may accelerate the rate of bodily defenses.

The degree of fever provides some rough estimate of the severity of infection. But it is only a crude estimate: for example, there is no significant difference between a fever of 101° or 102° F. One may also be quite sick without having appreciable fever, as is often true of patients with hepatitis, who may have liver inflammation, be quite jaundiced, and yet have normal body temperature. In describing a fever one should specify whether oral or rectal temperatures were taken. Normal rectal temperature is about 99.6° F., or one degree higher than normal mouth temperature, despite the fact that both kinds of thermometers indicate the normal at 98.6° F.

142

Whatever the value of fever, people with markedly elevated temperatures generally feel better if it is lowered somewhat. Aspirin in the usual doses possesses the property of lowering fevers. For a bacterial infection one would, of course, want to use an antibiotic to cure the infection. For fever associated with viral infection (one against which an antibiotic will not work) aspirin still remains the most useful drug.

Another measure for reducing high fevers is an alcohol sponging. For the rare but severe fever produced by sunstroke or certain viral infections in which the temperature can go to 104°-105° F., rapid decreases in body temperature are in order. This reduction can be achieved by direct applications of ice, pouring cool to cold water over various bodily surfaces, or wrapping in a cool wet sheet. Fevers of lesser magnitude generally present no emergency and do not call for heroic measures designed to beat the temperature down a degree or two. Moderate fever may be regarded as a help, not a hindrance, to bodily defenses. (See also TEMPERATURE, TAKING.)

FIBROID   A fibroid is a benign tumor occurring in the heavy muscular wall of the uterus. As is also true of tumors elsewhere, we do not know why fibroid tumors develop as often as they do. More than half of all women develop fibroids of some size. The tumors are frequently multiple and vary from marble-sized to orange-sized and even larger. Stimulation by the hormones produced by the ovary may increase their size. When there is a drop-off in ovarian hormones fibroid tumors may shrink, an event frequently seen after the menopause.

Because of the stimulating effect of hormones, fibroids may increase in size in women taking hormone injections or birth-control pills and also, for the same reason, during a normal pregnancy. Fibroids often reach larger size without producing any symptoms of any kind. In the absence of symptoms even a large uterine fibroid does not need to be removed. The difficulties produced by fibroids are the following: (1) Pressure symptoms—large fibroids can exert pressure on nearby organs such as the bladder and the rectum. The symptoms produced will be those of frequent urination, small bladder capacity, or difficulties in bowel function. (2) Abnormal bleeding may be produced by fibroids, with patterns of increased flow or more frequent menstruation; anemia may then result. (3) In some instances fibroids may contribute to sterility, either by interfering with conception or with the progress of pregnancy. (4) Sometimes because of impaired blood supply or for other reasons a fibroid may undergo degenerative changes and produce pain and fever.

Treatment. The treatment of fibroids must necessarily be very individualized. The doctor will want to be sure that there is no other associated condition producing abnormal symptoms. Up to a point it is possible to live with fibroids that are producing symptoms. Beyond this point surgery is often recommended. Complete removal of the uterus is the operation called hysterectomy. In younger women who still want to have children and where there is a reasonable chance that they may become pregnant, a surgical procedure known as a myomectomy may be performed instead. In such a case the surgeon will try to remove the fibroids alone, to the extent that this is possible, hoping to spare the uterus for further functioning. However, it is not always possible to do a myomectomy. Since fibroids tend to shrink after the menopause, a woman approaching it may sometimes put up with symptoms due to fibroids in the hope that spontaneous improvement will occur.

FIRST AID

The following 32-page *Emergency First Aid Guide* (adapted from a United States Government publication) presents instructions for use in a wide variety of emergency situations. Other emergency and medical problems are discussed throughout the text in more detail.

Use this handy First Aid Guide for instant answers to emergency questions.

Call a physician immediately for serious injuries, poisoning, and drug overdoses.

Instant Emergency
First Aid Guide

Index

Acid poisoning, 151
Alkali poisoning, 151
Animal bites, 169
Apoplexy-Stroke, 174
Artificial Respiration, 21, 149
Back, broken, 141
Bandaging, 168
Bites, animal, 169
Bites, insect, 154
Bites, snake, 152
Bleeding, 146
Blisters, 171
Bones, broken, 141
Breath stoppage, 21, 149
Bruises, 166
Burns, 156
Chemical burns, 153
Choking (on food), 161
Cold injuries, 162
Cut artery, 146
Cut vein, 146
Dislocations, 164
Electrical burns, 159
Epilepsy, the Seizure, 176
Excessive heat, 159
Exposure to cold, 162
Eye injuries, 169
Fainting, 175
Food poisoning, 151
Fractures, 141

Frostbite, 162
Gases, 149
Heart failure, 173
Heat exhaustion, 160
Heat injuries, 156
Infected wounds, 171
Injuries due to cold, 162
Insect stings, 154
Medical emergencies, 172
Nosebleed, 147
Objects under nails, 170
Objects under skin, 170
Poisoning, 150
Poisonous snakes, 152
Pressure points, 146
Puncture wounds, 168
Scalds, 156
Scorpion bites, 155
Shock, 148
Snake bite, 152
Snow blindness, 163
Spider bites, 155
Spine fracture, 141
Sprains, 165
Stings, 154
Stoppage of breath, 21, 149
Strains, 166
Sunburn, 159
Sunstroke, 159
Wounds, 167

Also, see regular index at the end of the book for more complete information on these and other emergencies.

SERIOUS BLEEDING

Cut Artery or Vein

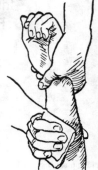

Symptoms

1. Cut artery, bright red blood spurts or wells up

2. Cut vein, dark red blood flows steadily or oozes

First Aid (Also see pp. 47, 49)

1. Remove or cut clothing from wound.

2. *Always apply pressure at once.* Seconds count. Loss of 2 pints of blood can be fatal.

    a. Apply direct firm pressure over wound with a sterile or clean dressing, or even your hand. Raise bleeding part if no bones broken.

    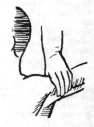

    b. If this fails to stop flow, apply firm strong pressure to nearest pressure point. See sketches.

    c. A constricting band should only be used for cut arteries that cannot be controlled by a. or b.

    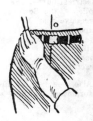

Internal Bleeding

Symptoms

1. Restlessness
2. Anxiety
3. Thirst
4. Pale face
5. Weak, rapid pulse
6. Weakness

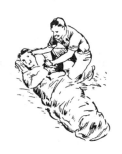

First Aid (Also see pp. 45, 49, 67)

1. Keep victim flat on back. Exception: If he cannot breathe because of chest injury.
2. Turn his head to side for vomiting.
3. Keep him quiet, reassured.
4. Move him only in lying position to a hospital.

Nose Bleed (Also see p. 47)

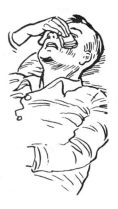

1. Have victim sit with head thrown back, breathing through mouth, clothing at neck loosened.
2. Press nostril continuously to middle portion for 5 to 10 minutes. This will stop nearly all bleeding in front of the nasal bones.
3. If bleeding continues pack gauze into nostril and take victim to doctor.

SHOCK

SHOCK is a depressed state of body functions caused by injury. Unless treated, the condition often results in death, although the injury itself would not be fatal.

TREAT FOR SHOCK IN ANY INJURY CASE

Factors Contributing to Shock

1. Exposure
2. Pain
3. Rough handling
4. Improper transportation
5. Loss of blood
6. Fatigue
7. Broken bones and internal injuries

Symptoms

1. Symptoms usually develop gradually and may not be noticeable at first
2. Skin pale, cold, moist, clammy
3. Eyes vacant, lackluster, pupils dilated
4. Breathing shallow, irregular; air hunger
5. Nausea, faintness, or even unconsciousness
6. Pulse weak, irregular, rapid, or absent in extreme cases

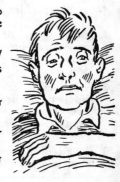

148

First Aid

1. Position: Keep victim lying flat. Raise legs 12 to 18 inches unless head or chest is injured.

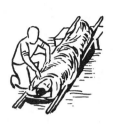

2. Heat: Keep victim only warm enough to prevent shivering. Conserve body heat by blanket underneath.

3. Fluids: If conscious, give water or dilute salt-soda solution (½ teaspoon of table salt and ½ teaspoon of baking soda to quart of water) as tolerated.

STOPPAGE OF BREATH

(CHOKING—See p. 161)
Smoke, Gases, Drowning, Electric Shock, Poisoning, or Nerve Injury.

Manual Method of Artificial Respiration (Use if mouth-to-mouth cannot be used) (Also see p. 22)

1. Place victim on back with support under shoulder to allow head to drop backward.

2. Kneel above victim's head, facing him.

3. Grasp his wrists, cross them and press them against the lower chest.

4. Immediately pull arms up, out, and back as far as possible.

5. Repeat 12–16 times per minute.

POISONING BY MOUTH

Objectives

To dilute the poison as fast as possible. Then except as advised induce vomiting.

Symptoms

1. Information from victim or observer, telltale container or sudden illness in well person
2. Odor of poison on breath
3. Mouth may be burned
4. Convulsions or unconsciousness

First Aid: Call doctor or hospital for instructions, or do as follows: (Also see pp. 244-246)

Poisons not Acid or Alkali

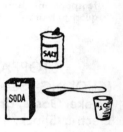

1. DILUTE: Give 4 or more glasses of milk or water.
2. Induce vomiting: Give glass of water containing several teaspoons of salt or baking soda; or induce gagging with finger or spoon. Repeat until you believe poison is washed out.
3. Give antidote, if one is known.
4. When poison is unknown give antidote of 1 part strong tea, 1 part milk of magnesia, 2 parts burnt toast.
5. Take to doctor—take poison container or vomitus for analysis.
6. If petroleum products, don't induce vomiting—dilute only.

Acids

1. Avoid vomiting if possible.
2. Neutralize with alkali such as baking soda, magnesia, chalk in water.
3. Give milk, olive oil, or egg white.

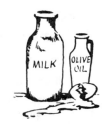

Alkalies

1. Avoid vomiting if possible.
2. Neutralize with weak acid such as lemon juice or vinegar.
3. Give milk.

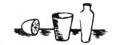

Skin Contamination

1. Drench with water.
2. Apply stream of water on skin while removing clothing.
3. Cleanse skin thoroughly again with water. Rapidity in washing is most important in reducing extent of injury.

Food Poisoning

Symptoms

1. Uncomfortable feeling in upper abdomen
2. Pain and cramps
3. Nausea and vomiting
4. Diarrhea

5. Prostration

6. Unconsciousness in severe cases

First Aid

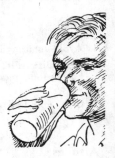

1. Call doctor.

2. Save samples of food, vomitus, or excreta for analysis.

3. Keep victim warm, in bed.

4. May give him sweetened strong tea or water as tolerated.

POISON SNAKES, INSECTS, PLANTS
(Also see p. 45)

SNAKE BITES. Only 10–20 deaths in U.S. every year. Only 2% of poisonous bites fatal.

Prevention

1. Wear high shoes.

2. Watch for snakes.

3. Carry snakebite kit.

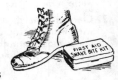

4. Differentiate poisonous snakes with typical fang punctures and nonpoisonous variety with multiple teeth marks. Coral snake is exception.

Symptoms

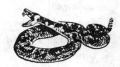

1. Immediate pain

2. Swelling, purple color

3. 1 or 2 fang puncture points

4. Weakness, short breath

5. Rapid, weak pulse

6. Vomiting, faintness

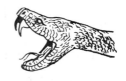

First Aid

1. Apply a constricting band above the injury. Apply cold packs and transport immediately to the nearest hospital or doctor.

2. If professional help is not available within a few hours—

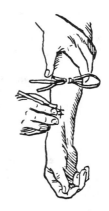

   a. Apply constricting band above bitten part or area of swelling. Loosen every 15 minutes for a few seconds.

   b. Sterilize a knife or razor blade over match flame.

   c. Make half-inch cuts through fang marks parallel to limb.

   d. Any cross cuts should be very shallow to avoid injury to nerves or tendons, especially in hand or wrist.

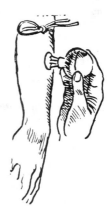

   e. Apply suction by bulb or mouth (Venom is not a stomach poison but rinse mouth if gums are cut or infected).

f. Continue suction for at least 1 hour—little value after this.

g. If area of swelling moves, move band and repeat cuts and suction.

h. Give fluids as desired. No alcohol.

i. Keep victim quiet and warm.

j. Apply cold compresses to swelling and transport victim, with part down, to doctor.

k. In isolated areas employees should be trained to use antivenim.

l. Treat nonpoisonous snake bites like any other wound.

Insect Sting—Bee or Wasp (Also see pp. 43-44)

Persons sensitive to insect stings should get vaccine before insect season.

1. Remove stinger if possible. (Honey bee)

2. Apply paste of baking soda and cold cream.

3. Cold applications will relieve pain.

4. Calamine lotion will relieve itching.

5. If unusual reaction, or history of a severe reaction, apply constricting band above bite, cold packs and rush to doctor.

Black Widow Spider and Scorpion Bites
(Also see p. 44)

Symptoms

1. Slight swelling, redness

2. Immediate burning, spreading pain

3. Abdominal pain and rigidity, nausea and vomiting

4. Fever, sweating, severe headache

5. Rarely fatal in adults

First Aid

1. Keep victim lying down, quiet and warm.

2. Apply constricting band above bite and loosen every 15 minutes.

3. Apply cold pack over bite.

4. Take to doctor.

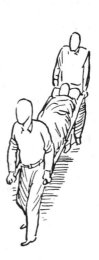

HEAT INJURIES

Burns and Scalds

Symptoms and Classification

1. First degree—skin reddened

2. Second degree—skin blistered

3. Third degree—skin cooked or charred, may extend to underlying tissue

First Aid

For small first and second degree burns covering up to 1 percent of body surface (size of hand):

1. Wash gently with soap and water.

2. If ice water is available, soak the part 20 to 30 minutes.

3. If skin is broken may use approved antiseptic.

4. Place sterile or clean gauze over burned area.

5. Bandage entire area snugly.

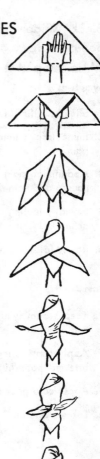

For large second and third degree burns:

1. If doctor or hospital is available:

   a. Cover with sterile or clean dressing.

   b. Treat for shock.

   c. Rush to hospital.

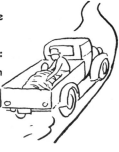

2. If in isolated area:

   a. Remove clothing from burn, cut around cloth that sticks to burned area.

   b. May apply approved antiseptic.

   c. Cover burn with sterile dressing.

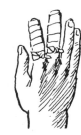

   d. Cover this with 8 to 10 layers of loose sterile or clean dressing.

   e. Dress burn so it cannot touch other burned or unburned skin.

   f. Bandage snugly so there is moderate pressure on burn.

   g. Treat for shock.

   h. If victim is conscious, he should drink all he wishes of solution containing 1/2 teaspoon baking soda and 1/2 teaspoon of salt to 1 quart of water.

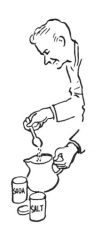

157

i. **DO NOT**

    (1) Touch burn with fingers.

    (2) Breathe on burn.

    (3) Apply antiseptic other than as indicated above.

    (4) Break or drain blisters.

    (5) Change dressing. Doctor should do this.

Chemical Burns

1. Flush thoroughly with water to remove all of chemical.

2. Treat like other burns.

3. If eye is burned hold eyelid open and flush with water, cover with sterile compress and get to doctor.

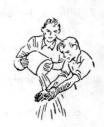

Inhalation Burns

1. Carry patient to fresh air immediately.

2. Apply artificial respiration if breathing has stopped or is inadequate.

3. Prevent chilling.

4. Do not give alcohol in any form.

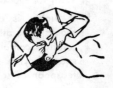

Electric Burns

Treat like other burns, but cover wider area with dressing because these burns are usually more extensive than they appear to be.

Sunburn

Use petrolatum or cold cream for mild cases. For severe sunburn treat as other burns.

Excessive Heat

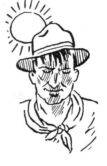

Some of the adverse effects of excessive heat and copious sweating may be lessened by the regular use of ample drinking water and liberally salted foods, rarely salt tablets.

Sunstroke

Cause

Exposure to heat, particularly the sun's rays

Symptoms

1. Headache
2. Dizziness
3. Red face
4. Hot, dry skin

5. Strong, rapid pulse

6. Very high temperature

7. Usually unconscious

First Aid

1. Put victim in shade, lying on back, with head and shoulders raised, clothing removed.

2. Cool the body with ice, water or "rubbing alcohol" or fanning.

3. Give cool drinks, no stimulants.

4. Call doctor.

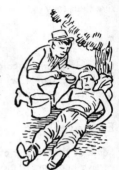

Heat Exhaustion
(Also see pp. 199-200)

Cause

Exposure to heat either outdoors or indoors.

Symptoms

1. Pale face

2. Dizziness

3. Vomiting

4. Profuse sweating

5. Moist cool skin

6. Weak pulse

7. Low temperature

8. Faint but seldom unconscious for long

9. May have cramps in abdomen or limbs

First Aid

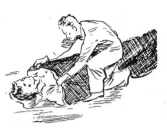

1. Lay victim down with body level or head slightly lowered.

2. Give several glasses of solution of 1/2 teaspoon salt in glass of water.

3. Remove victim to circulating air and out of direct sun rays.

Choking (Food lodged in windpipe)

Symptoms

1. Unable to speak or breathe.
2. May be unconscious.
3. Skin turns blue.

First Aid

1. Stand behind the person and put your arms around him.
2. Make a fist with one hand.
3. Grasp your fist with the other hand, pressing at a spot above the navel and below the ribs.
4. With a quick, upward thrust, expel the object. Repeat if necessary.

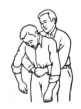

If you see someone choking, don't wait. There are only four minutes from the time the victim starts choking to the time of brain damage or death.

INJURIES DUE TO COLD

Frost Bite

Symptoms

1. Considerable pain and redness in fingers, toes, cheeks, ears, or nose

2. Later grayish-white color due to frozen tissues

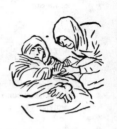

First Aid

1. Until victim can be brought indoors, cover part with woolen cloth or warm skin of victim or first aider.

2. Thaw out frozen part rapidly in warm room, or in warm water 100°–105° F. or electric blankets at 100° F.

3. Encourage movement of part.

4. Apply dry sterile or clean dressing.

5. May give warm drinks.

6. Get early medical attention.

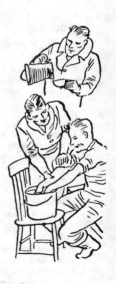

Prolonged Exposure to Cold

Symptoms

1. Victim becomes numb, drowsy

2. He staggers, eyesight fails, and he becomes unconscious

First Aid

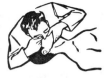

1. Place him in warm room and apply artificial respiration if breathing has stopped.

2. If only chilled and not unconscious, put him in warm bed and give hot drinks.

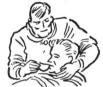

Snow Blindness

Prevention

Wear good quality, dark glasses in snow country, particularly in early spring and at high elevations.

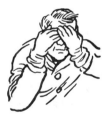

Symptoms

1. Burning, smarting, sandy feeling in eyes

2. Pain in eyes or forehead

3. Sensitivity to light, eyes watering

First Aid

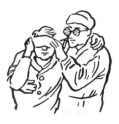

1. Cold compresses on eyes.

2. Use mild eye drops or mineral oil.

   Wear dark glasses.

DISLOCATIONS, SPRAINS, STRAINS, BRUISES

Dislocations

Symptoms

1. Intense pain

2. Deformity

3. Swelling

4. Loss of movement

First Aid

1. Treat as fracture.

2. If necessary to move victim, support dislocated elbow or shoulder in loose sling; if hip dislocated, place pillow under knees.

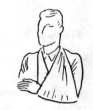

3. Gentle traction may be tried to reduce the dislocation of finger joints. If it fails, do not persist. This should not be tried for a dislocated thumb.

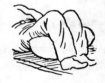

4. Apply cold and transport to doctor.

Sprain

SPRAINS ARE TEARS OF LIGAMENTS SUPPORTING A JOINT

Symptoms

1. Pain at joint

2. Swelling

3. Discoloring

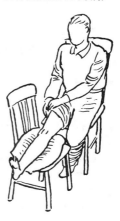

First Aid

1. Elevate the part, if practical, by putting wrist in sling, ankle on pillows.

2. Apply cold applications or ice packs to reduce swelling and pain; hot applications after 24 hours.

3. All sprains should be X-rayed for possible fracture.

4. If person must walk with sprained ankle, support it as shown in the sketch.

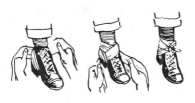

Strains

STRAINS ARE INJURIES TO MUSCLES OR TENDONS

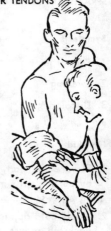

Symptoms

Pain in muscles, increasing stiffness

First Aid

1. Rest injured muscle.
2. In first 24 hours, cold packs to relieve pain and avoid swelling.
3. After 24 hours, heat to reduce muscle spasm and increase circulation.
4. Massage to loosen up muscles.

Bruises

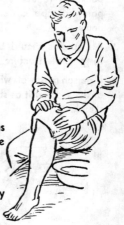

Symptoms

Pain, swelling, discoloration

First Aid

1. Apply ice packs or cold cloths to reduce swelling and relieve pain.
2. Elevate injured part.
3. If skin is broken, treat as any open wound.

WOUNDS AND BANDAGING

ALL WOUNDS, NO MATTER
HOW SMALL, SHOULD BE
TREATED TO PREVENT INFEC-
TION. WHEN BLEEDING IS
NOT SEVERE, INFECTION IS THE
CHIEF DANGER. UNCLEAN
FIRST AID IS MORE DANGER-
OUS THAN NO TREATMENT AT
ALL.

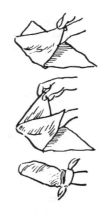

First Aid

1. If wound is severe and doctor
   is nearby, cover wound with
   sterile pad, then bandage and
   take victim to doctor.

2. In isolated areas, if possible
   thoroughly wash wound with
   soap and water; then cover with
   sterile pad and bandage.
   Otherwise cover and bandage
   until washing can be done later.

3. If wound is so large that it will
   have to be sewed up:

   a. After washing, cover with
      sterile gauze, then bandage
      and take victim to doctor.

   b. If doctor cannot be reached
      for several hours, after wash-
      ing, close wound by finger

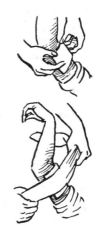

pressure and apply butterfly taping, then bandage.

4. If wound is well washed, no antiseptic is needed. If one is used, povidone-iodine complex is suggested.

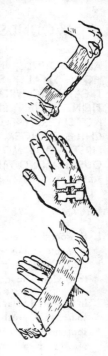

Bandaging

1. Always apply sterile gauze pad directly on wound, then bandage over this.

2. Never use absorbent cotton or adhesive tape directly on a wound, except a narrow bridge of adhesive, sterilized over flame, to hold wound edges together.

3. Bandage snugly but not tightly; ends of fingers and toes uncovered, if possible, to check on circulation.

Puncture Wound

1. Encourage bleeding by mild pressure at edge of wound.

2. Wash with soap and water.

3. May apply approved antiseptic.

4. Apply sterile pad and bandage.

5. Doctor should determine need for tetanus vaccine.

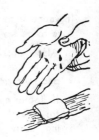

Animal Bite (Also see p. 43)

Dog, Cat, Wildlife, Any Mammal

1. Wash wound thoroughly with soap and water.

2. Apply sterile pad and bandage.

3. Consult doctor about rabies or tetanus shots.

4. Confine animal for observation. If necessary to kill, do not damage its brain, so that it may be examined.

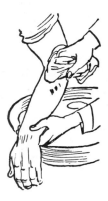

Eye Wound (Also see pp. 138-141)

Object imbedded in eye or surrounding tissues:

1. Do not permit victim to rub the eye.

2. Pull down lower lid to remove object with clean handkerchief or grasp edge of upper lid, make slight pressure on the skin surface of the lid with the side of a blunt pencil or the edge of a match stick, and turn the inner surface of the lid upward and remove object.

3. If the foreign body is seen on the clear front part of the eye have patient wink several times and see if it can be dislodged.

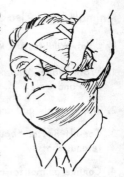

4. If the foreign body is imbedded and cannot be dislodged do not attempt to remove it. Have the patient close the eye, place a pad or piece of moist cotton over the closed lid, bandage and obtain medical attention.

Objects under Skin and Nails

1. Wash part with soap and water.

2. Sterilize needle, knife, or tweezers in flame, then remove object.

3. Encourage bleeding by gentle pressure.

4. May apply approved antiseptic.

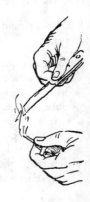

5. Apply sterile pad and bandage.

6. If splinter breaks off under nail, scrape nail thin, then cut V-piece over splinter, remove as above, if patient cannot be taken to doctor within 12 hours.

Blisters (Also see pp. 65, 73)

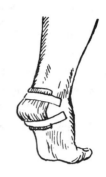

1. Wash with soap and warm water.
2. Sterilize needle over open flame.
3. Puncture blister at edge.
4. Gently press out water or blood with sterile pad.
5. May apply approved antiseptic.
6. Apply sterile dressing.
7. If blister develops infection see doctor.
8. Small blisters — merely wash and cover with sterile bandage; only puncture when large and must to get shoe on, etc.

Infected Wounds

Symptoms

1. Throbbing pain and heat
2. Extreme swelling, redness
3. Pus and red streaks
4. Tenderness, fever
5. Swollen glands

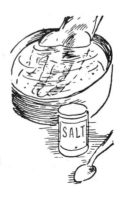

First Aid

1. Rest in bed or rest infected part.

2. Soak part in warm salt solution (2 teaspoons salt to quart of water) for 30 minutes.

3. Or, apply warm moist packs (same solution), wrung dry.

4. Repeat every few hours until medical attention.

5. Between soaks elevate and apply sterile dressing.

MEDICAL EMERGENCIES

Insulin Reaction—Diabetics
(Also see p. 108)

Symptoms (usually sudden onset)

1. Skin—moist and pale

2. Rapid pulse

3. Tremor or even convulsions

4. Victim becomes weak; may become unconscious

First Aid

1. If conscious, give sugar, candy, or orange juice.

2. If unconscious, get to doctor for injection.

Heart Attack (Also see p. 55)

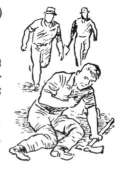

Symptoms

1. Pain—heavy and excruciating under the breastbone; may radiate to neck, jaws or arms; may be in upper abdomen

2. Shortness of breath, may feel he has to sit, stand, or walk to breathe

3. May perspire freely

4. May be in shock

5. Often severe anxiousness

6. Often history of previous bouts of pain behind the breastbone, especially with exertion

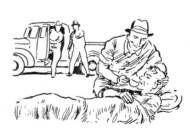

First Aid

1. Call doctor.

2. If victim has medication for pain have him take it.

3. Put at rest and make comfortable.

4. Give oxygen if available.

5. Stay with him and reduce his anxiety.

6. Treat shock.

7. Transport only if necessary—preferably lying down with head level (head down in cases of shock).

Apoplexy-Stroke (Also see pp. 18, 55)

APOPLEXY OR STROKE RESULTS FROM RUPTURE OF A BLOOD VESSEL IN THE BRAIN OR A BLOOD CLOT

Symptoms

1. May follow over-exertion

2. Face may be red, but sometimes ashen gray

3. Slow pulse and heavy breathing

4. One eye pupil may be larger than other

5. One side of body may be paralyzed or victim may have difficulty speaking

6. May be unconscious

7. May be very minor, especially in older persons, with only headache and dizziness; sudden memory loss, change of mood, numbness or difficulty using body part.

First Aid

1. Lay victim on back with head and shoulders raised.
2. Nothing by mouth unless fully conscious.
3. Keep warm and comfortable.
4. Call doctor.
5. If doctor is not available, transport lying down with head raised.

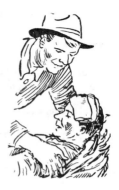

Fainting (Also see p. 141)

Prevention

Victim should sit down and put head between knees, or lie down immediately.

Symptoms

1. Pale face, drooping eyelids
2. Perspiration
3. Dizzy
4. Shallow breathing
5. Weak pulse
6. Unconsciousness finally

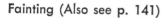

First Aid

1. Keep victim lying down, with head lower than body.
2. Loosen tight clothing.
3. Can use ammonia inhalant.
4. Keep him resting until fully recovered.

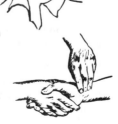

Epilepsy (Also see p. 233)

Symptoms

1. Convulsion may or may not come with warning

2. Pale face, eyes roll up

3. Victim utters hoarse cry, falls to ground

4. Turns blue, bites tongue, loses consciousness

5. Jerks head, arms, legs wildly

6. Froths at mouth

7. May become conscious, or else pass into deep sleep in 2 to 30 minutes

First Aid

1. Prevent victim injuring himself by pushing objects out of the way.

2. If anticipated, place soft object between teeth.

3. Let victim rest undisturbed after attack. Do all you can to keep embarrassment at a minimum.

FORMULA

▶ **Kinds and Amounts** Most babies thrive on very simple formulas. Formulas are usually mixtures of cow's milk, water, and sugar. As a baby grows older, water and sugar are gradually cut down until he is taking milk alone.

Your doctor will tell you how to make your baby's formula and how to change it from time to time. However, if you are unable to get in touch with your doctor, a formula that suits most young babies is:

Evaporated milk ....4 ounces
Water ....8 ounces
Sugar ....1 tablespoon (level)
    or
Whole milk ....8 ounces
Water ....4 ounces
Sugar ....1 tablespoon (level)

This mixture may be divided into 6 bottles of about 2 ounces each or eight bottles of about 1½ ounces each. This amount of feeding usually satisfies a newborn baby from about the second or third day to the end of the first week.

As soon as your baby is no longer satisfied with this amount of feeding, double the amounts in the original formula. Later, when the baby wants it, use 3 times the amount of each item in the formula.

Most babies do well if they are given as much of this milk mixture as they wish when they are hungry, which will usually be about every 3 to 4 hours. After your baby is 2 weeks old he will need in each 24 hours from 2 to 3 ounces of this milk mixture for each pound that he weighs. If in 24 hours your baby usually takes less than 2 ounces of this formula for each pound that he weighs, tell your doctor about that.

A formula which has less water in it may be quite satisfactory for your baby, particularly when he is 2 or 3 months old. Gradually cut down the amount of water until he is taking whole milk or until he is taking equal parts of evaporated milk and water.

When your baby is taking other foods, it is time to stop adding sugar to the milk. If sugar is cut down slowly, your baby will probably not miss it. (See also INFANT FEEDING.)

In general, there are two simple ways of making a formula

safe for a baby. The first way is to mix the formula, pour it, unboiled, into bottles that have been washed but not sterilized, put on the nipples, and last, sterilize the filled bottles. The second method is to sterilize the equipment, boil the formula, and then pour the boiled milk into the sterilized bottles. Either way is all right. You can, if you like, try both ways and see which seems simpler to you.

▶ **Feeding Equipment** The standard-sized nursing bottle holds 8 ounces. Lines are marked where the ounces come, so there need be no guesswork when you pour in the formula. Bottles of heat-resistant glass or of boilable plastic cost more, but you will probably save in the long run by getting them. Buy bottles that are easy to clean with a bottle brush. The neck of the bottle as well as the bottom should slope into the sides, so there are no sharp, hard-to-clean corners.

Buy as many bottles as you will need in a 24-hour period. A dozen will be none too many, and a few more will come in handy in case you break any. In addition to the number of bottles you use for feedings, you will need two or three for water and orange juice. These can be 4-ounce bottles. Bottles are easier to clean if you rinse them after each feeding and fill them with cold water.

If you can, buy enough nipples so that you will not have to boil them but once a day. This will mean having one for each feeding and one for each drink of water or orange juice. You may have to make the holes in the nipples larger. Try out the nipples by putting one on a bottle with water in it and turning it upside down. Watch to see if there is a steady drip. Remember that water will come through faster than milk because it is thinner.

If the holes seem too small, heat the point of a fine needle in the flame of a match. While the point is red hot, poke it quickly through one or more holes in the nipple. Be sure to use a small needle as it is easy to ruin a nipple by burning too large holes in it. After each feeding, wash the nipple and squeeze water through the holes. Dry it and keep it in a covered jar until you are ready to sterilize the day's supply.

Nipple caps or covers are made of glass, plastic, aluminum, or paper. Paper caps are the cheapest, but since they can be used only once, they may not be the most economical in the long run.

▶ **Equipment for Making**   It is convenient to have a set of utensils that you use only in preparing your baby's food. In any case, keeping utensils together will make the sterilizing and formula preparation go more speedily.

Kettle for sterilizing. If you are going to bottle-feed a baby for a long time, it may pay you to buy a kettle specially made for this purpose. Such a kettle has a tight-fitting cover and a rack inside to hold the bottles.

If you do not want to go to this expense, any kettle large enough to hold the bottles and other equipment will do. If you have a large enough pressure cooker, you can use it as a kettle.

In addition to the kettle you will need:

A wire rack or a pie tin (upside down) that fits the bottom of the kettle, for holding the bottles.

A bottle brush with a long handle and with stout bristles to scrub the inside of the bottles. It should be one that is bent at the tip so that the bristles clean the bottom of the bottle and not just the sides.

A set of measuring spoons is handy.

A measuring cup marked in ounces, with a pouring lip.

A 2-quart saucepan with a pouring lip to mix the formula in.

A small saucepan with a lid, in which to boil and keep the nipples.

A funnel makes it easier to pour the formula into the bottles, but if your saucepan has a lip that pours well you may be able to get along without one. If you get a plastic one, make sure it is the kind which can be boiled.

A long-handled spoon.

A can opener that punches holes (if you use canned milk).

A small wide-mouthed jar with a cover, for used nipples.

Bottles to hold a 24-hour supply of formula.

Nipples and nipple caps.

A pair of tongs is convenient.

▶ **Making the Formula—Method I (Terminal Sterilization)**
1. Wash thoroughly with hot water and detergent all the articles you will use. With the bottle brush scrub the inside of the bottles and nipple covers and the inside and outside of the nipples.
2. Rinse all articles well. Drain. Squeeze clean water through nipple holes.

3. Measure the milk, water, and sugar or syrup into a large saucepan. If you use granulated sugar, level off measuring spoon with back of table knife. If you use syrup, pour from the bottle into the measuring spoon. If the milk you use is not homogenized, shake the bottle well to mix the cream before measuring. If you use evaporated milk, wash the top of the can with soap and water and rinse it off well before opening.

4. Divide the milk mixture among the number of bottles the baby is likely to need in 24 hours.

5. Put nipples and nipple covers on the bottles. Do not push or screw nipple covers down tight, because during sterilization the hot air may blow the caps off.

6. Put the bottles of formula on the rack in the kettle. Put one or two bottles of drinking water, covered with nipple and cap, in at the same time. Pour water into the kettle until it comes about halfway up on the bottle. Cover the kettle.

7. Bring the water in the kettle to a boil. *Boil actively for 25 minutes* by the clock. As soon as the bottles cool enough to handle, take them out of the kettle. Tighten nipple caps.

8. After the bottles cool, put them in your refrigerator at once. In an ice refrigerator, place the bottles near the ice. A rack to hold the bottles upright is very convenient.

▶ **Method II (Standard Clean Technique)** *Sterilizing the equipment.* You may like to sterilize ahead of the time when you make the formula. Then the things in the sterilizing kettle will have a chance to cool down before you need to handle them in making the formula.

1. Wash the bottles, nipple covers, funnel and nipples thoroughly in hot water with a detergent. With the bottle brush scrub the inside of the nursing bottles and nipple covers, and inside and outside of the nipples.

2. Rinse all these articles well. Squeeze clean water through the nipple holes.

3. If your sterilizing kettle has a rack to hold the bottles, set each bottle in it, upside down. Fit the other articles between the bottles. If your kettle has no rack, lay the bottles on their sides in the kettle, with the other equipment on top.

4. If your kettle has a rack and a tight-fitting cover, pour in 1 or 2 inches of water and put on the cover. When the water boils actively, steam will form and will sterilize the

equipment. Keep the water boiling for at least 5 minutes by the clock. If your kettle doesn't have a tight-fitting lid, put in enough water to completely cover the bottles and all the other things to be sterilized. Boil for at least 5 minutes after the water has come to a boil.

5. If you put enough water in the kettle to cover the bottles and other articles, they will cool more quickly if you drain off some of the water. Leave the things in the covered kettle until ready to use.

6. Drop the nipples into boiling water in a small pan, cover, and let boil for 5 minutes. Then pour the water off, let the steam escape and leave the nipples in the covered pan until you use them.

Sterilizing the formula.

1. Measure the milk, water, and sugar or syrup into a large saucepan. To make up for water lost during boiling you can put in an ounce or so more water than your formula calls for. If you use granulated sugar, level off measuring spoon with back of table knife. If you use syrup, pour from the bottle into the measuring spoon. If the milk you use is not homogenized, shake the bottle well to mix the cream before measuring. If you use evaporated milk, wash the top of the can with soap and water and rinse it off well before opening it.

2. Bring the mixture to a boil and keep boiling (bubbling) gently for 5 minutes by the clock. Stir constantly with a large stirring spoon.

3. Take the milk mixture off the stove and let it cool for a few minutes. Stirring it will make it cool faster. If you use fresh milk, stirring will keep scum from forming.

4. Take the nursing bottles out of the sterilizer without touching the tops, using tongs if you have them. If you use a funnel take it out of the sterilizer without touching its rim or stem, and set it in one of the bottles.

5. Divide the milk mixture among the number of bottles the baby is likely to need in 24 hours.

6. Put sterile rubber nipples on the bottles without touching the rim of the bottle or the nipple except by the tab or outer edge. Cover the nipples at once with sterile nipple caps, being careful not to touch nipples or lip of nipple caps. (Follow the directions that come with whatever kind of nipple and bottle you use.)

7. Put the bottles in the refrigerator at once. In an ice refrigerator, place the bottles near the ice.

GALLBLADDER, DISEASES OF   The gallbladder is roughly comparable in size and shape to a small pear. It is located in the upper right quarter of the abdomen. Its location can be approximated as being in the area where a line dropped from the right nipple meets the lowermost rib. The pain of gallbladder disease is most often felt in this location. In addition, it may also be felt at approximately the same point in the back and occasionally in the tip of the right shoulder.

The movement of stones out of the gallbladder—termed biliary colic—may produce paroxysms of intense pain which radiate to the upper central abdomen. Gallstones may vary from the size of a pinhead to that of a marble, and will develop at one time or another in 10 to 20 per cent of the population. They may or may not be associated with inflammation of the gallbladder itself, and may or may not produce symptoms.

Acute inflammation of the gallbladder, known as *cholecystitis,* usually comes on suddenly. It produces pain in the region of the gallbladder, often accompanied by nausea and vomiting and a variable degree of fever. It may be mild and subside, or severe, in which case, like acute appendicitis, rupture and peritonitis may result. Hence, depending on the course of events, it may be allowed to subside or urgent operation may be necessary. It may occur in bouts weeks to years apart, and is often associated with gallstones. The acute disorder may give way to a chronic one in which there are many repeated bouts of pain in the right upper abdomen with bloating and nausea, often brought on by dietary indiscretions such as eating certain fats.

Gallbladder disease is often regarded as a surgical and not a medical disorder, for the following reasons: (1) Once any sort of gallbladder disorder, be it acute inflammation or colic, has occurred, repeated attacks can be expected. (2) There is no known medical treatment which will do away with gallstones once they have formed. (3) It is easier on both patient and surgeon to remove a diseased gallbladder at a time other than that of an acute attack, even though the patient has to be persuaded to be operated on when he is well, not sick. Exceptions to the rule of surgery may occur if the patient is old and in poor physical condition, if one or two large stones are found on an X-ray but no symptoms are referable to them, or if a long period has passed since an attack without any evidence of progression.

During an acute attack of gallbladder disease the usual treatment will consist of strict food abstinence (though fluids are occasionally permitted) and pain-killing drugs. Where bacterial infection is suspected, antibiotics (tetracyclines) may be given.

Gallstones, common in adults, do occur in children, but only rarely as part of a disease called cholelithiasis. Cholelithiasis is sometimes seen in congenital hemolytic anemia and sickle-cell anemia. In these conditions there is excess destruction of red blood cells, and the pigment released forms stones in the gallbladder. These may obstruct the gallbladder duct or cause inflammation. Jaundice may result and the gallbladder may have to be surgically removed.

GENES   The genes are the units of heredity. They can be looked upon as an exceedingly long list of directions which determine the structure and much of the functioning of the offspring. The enormous number of genes present in each of us is indicated when one reflects on the innumerable characteristics that are unique to one individual as compared to another: height; weight; eye, skin, and hair color; nose size; jaw formation; body build; sex; hair distribution; intelligence (I.Q.); and musical and mathematical abilities—not to mention all of the disorders or illnesses that have a family background, such as high blood pressure, diabetes, high blood cholesterol, gout, etc. Many thousands of messengers are obviously needed to transmit the appropriate instructions.

Recent investigations have indicated that the chemical messengers involved are highly specialized components of desoxyribonucleic acid (DNA) contained within the nucleus of the cell; various arrangements of molecules of nucleoprotein lead to various kinds of messages. All the genes are laid out in linear fashion on strands called chromosomes which become apparent under the microscope, particularly during the process of cell division. There are forty-six chromosomes in all of the cells in human beings, with one exception: only half this number is present in the sex cells, the ovum of the female and the sperm of the male. When the sperm fertilizes the egg, the twenty-three chromosomes of each sex cell are combined, thus restoring the count of forty-six in the fertilized egg. In usual cell division, which occurs countless times within the body in all of its growing tissues—such as the skin, the blood cells, or the lining of the intestines—the cell with forty-six chromosomes undergoes a reduplication of its chromosomes during division. This produces two daughter cells, each with the appropriate number of forty-six chromosomes.

There is one dissimilar pair of chromosomes found in males known as the XY pair. In females a corresponding pair of chromosomes known as XX is found. It is possible to take a few cells, as for example, blood cells or cells from the inner surface of the cheek, stain them, and (with the microscope) tell whether they came from a male or a female, because the XX pair of chromosomes produces a dot within the nucleus of the cell which is not found in males. It is of interest that the sex of the offspring is contributed by the male, not by the female. This occurs because half the male's sperm contain an X chromosome, half a Y chromosome, whereas all egg cells contain only an X chromosome. If an X-bearing sperm fertilizes the egg, the offspring will have an XX pair and be a female; if a Y-bearing sperm fertilizes it, the offspring is XY or male. Certain disorders associated with the X or Y chromosome are referred to as sex-linked. The most common are the varying degrees of baldness in the male which are transmitted on the X chromosome of the mother. Thus, baldness in a son can be anticipated from looking at the mother's brothers, not by looking at his father. (See also BALDNESS.)

Rare abnormalities referable to the XY pair of chromosomes may occur because of a failure to separate in the formation of the egg cell or the sperm cell. This can lead to odd and unusual combinations in which the offspring may have forty-seven or even more chromosomes, with combinations such as XXY, XXXY, and others. Some of these combinations are associated with defects in sex organ formation, infertility, short stature, and other deviations.

GENITAL HYGIENE, INFANT   The practice of cleaning the genital area is about the same as for other areas of the body. A daily bath with soap and water is desirable. In girl infants and little girls, the labia (lips) should be separated and the parts cleansed so that mucous secretions do not accumulate in the creases and folds. Uncircumcised boys should have the foreskin gently drawn back so that accumulations of mucus (smegma) may be removed. Thorough drying is advisable to prevent moisture accumulation with chafing and irritation of the skin. A lotion or talcum powder may be used to prevent irritating rashes in these areas.

GENITOURINARY DISEASES   Genitourinary infections are those which involve any areas of the urinary tract, the kidneys, bladder, and ureters (tubes leading from the kidney to the bladder carrying urine).

▶ **Pyelitis**   Symptoms of urinary tract infection may include abdominal pain, vomiting, diarrhea, back pain, fever, burning on urination, frequency of urination, urgency to urinate, and tenderness in the kidney area. Examination of the urine in this condition shows pus and bacteria in some specimens, with occasional casts and red blood cells. Treatment is with antibiotics. These infections may sometimes recur secondarily as a result of other, upper respiratory or generalized, systemic infections.

▶ **Postinfectious Hemorrhagic Nephritis**   This type of kidney infection frequently follows tonsillitis or other respiratory infections. It may be caused by a streptococcus. Ankle swelling, puffiness around the eyes, fever, pallor, malaise, with smoky or frankly bloody urine, may appear. Headache and other signs of high blood pressure may occur. Microscopic examination of the urine shows blood or albumin and casts. Treatment involves antibiotics, fluids, and other measures if complications occur. Most cases recover. If the condition progresses, it may develop into a chronic one.

▶ **Nephrosis**   Nephrosis is a kidney disease characterized by excess loss of albumin and proteins in the urine. Nephrosis causes swelling around the eyes, ankles, and in the abdomen. It is usually preceded by some infection. The urine shows large amounts of albumin, casts, and fatty substances. There may be high cholesterol in the blood. This is a chronic disease and extends over many years. Recent treatment with ACTH and steroids has improved the prognosis of this disease.

GROWTH AND DEVELOPMENT—CRITICAL NORMS

It is obvious that your child's stage of development will determine his ability to respond to your requirements and your demands upon him. The critical norms of development for parents to be aware of are listed below:

1. *Head control.* If your baby is unable to hold his head erect and steady without support by four months, there should be some investigation as to why he is unable to do this.

2. *Vision.* If the child does not follow objects moving across his line of vision by four months.

3. *Hearing.* If your child does not turn in the direction of a loud noise, say a telephone bell or a voice, by seven months.

4. *Grasping.* If your child does not reach out to grasp objects, hold them for several minutes, and/or transfer them from one hand to the other by seven months of age.

5. *Sitting.* If the infant does not sit up on a flat surface without support for a few minutes at a time by ten months of age.

6. *Babbling.* If your child does not make recognizable babbling sounds of two syllables, such as, "Dada," "Baba," "Mama," by ten months.

7. *Prehension.* If your child cannot grasp small objects with the thumb and index finger by ten months.

8. *Feeding.* If your child does not hold a glass and drink from it or use a spoon to feed himself by eighteen months.

9. *Walking.* If your child does not take steps across the room without support and without falling down by eighteen months.

10. *Speaking.* If your child does not use several words spontaneously and appropriately, that is, saying "milk" or "ball" upon seeing the object, by eighteen months.

11. *Climbing.* If your child does not try climbing on and off a chair, bed, or stair by twenty-four months.

12. *Sentences.* If your child does not speak in sentences by three years. A sentence is defined as two or more words which do not usually go together in a familiar phrase. "Baby wants ball" is a sentence.

If your infant or child fails to develop according to these general levels, a complete evaluation should be made by your physician or a neurologist.

GROWTH AND DEVELOPMENT—THE FIRST SIX MONTHS

Growth is increase in size. Development is increase in maturity and function. There are many factors which influence the normal development of a child, such as nationality, heredity, individuality, nutrition, endocrine factors, disease, environment, and social and economic conditions. There is, therefore, considerable variation in height, weight, and achievements at every age. The following are some of the average descriptions of babies.

1 Month. The baby moves his arms and legs at random and kicks aimlessly. He sucks, swallows, sneezes, and can generally put his fist, or sometimes a finger, into his mouth. He generally can look only straight ahead and not too much around him. If something is put into his hand he drops it fairly soon. His head generally sags a bit. He makes small noises, gurgles, and stares continuously at things around him. His eyes follow light but he cannot really focus or see too much.

2 Months. Real smiles of recognition may be seen and he will become more responsive. He may be able to gurgle and coo and listen to the sound of his own voice.

3 Months. He may develop head control while lying on his back.

4 Months. Usually the head will be steady while the baby is sitting and he can lift it up when he is on his stomach. His eyes will follow moving objects well, and his arms will start to move when he sees a toy. He will take the toy in his hand and/or put it to his mouth, and he looks at objects much more carefully. He may laugh out loud, become excited and show a spontaneous smile when greeted. He plays with things in his hand and he fingers objects. He follows moving objects with his eyes. There is some hand control at this time and his head can be kept still.

5 Months. He sometimes can roll back and forth on his abdomen and back and may turn over.

6 Months. He tries to sit up by himself.

GROWTH AND DEVELOPMENT—7 MONTHS TO 18 MONTHS

7 Months. He may sit up erect by himself, may

call, and may transfer objects from one hand to the other. At 7 months he has a one-hand approach and a grasp of toys. He may shake and bang a rattle and transfer a toy from one hand to the other. He may be able to put his toes into his mouth, make certain vowel sounds, and make noises called "vocalizing" when he is crying or babbling.

8 Months. He may be able to put his thumb and forefinger together, which is called prehension. This enables him to manipulate objects and toys that interest him.

9 Months. He may stand by himself or if held. He may bounce on standing.

10 Months. He may creep or crawl and sit up perfectly steadily by himself. He may pull himself to his feet at a rail. He may say "Mama" or "Dada," or one other word. He can probably feed himself a cracker or a piece of something and hold his own bottle.

11 Months. He may walk with or without support, or simply pull himself up to a standing position and remain standing for some time.

12 Months. He may walk with or without support. He may stand alone. He plays with objects and may say "Mama" and "Dada," and he sometimes will give a toy on request and cooperate in dressing.

16 to 18 Months. He climbs, runs, and develops some small skills with toys. He may turn the pages of a book or put blocks in a hole. He may use a spoon. He may say a few words. He may discard the bottle and indicate when he is wet.

18 Months. He usually walks without falling, turns the pages of a book, may build a tower of three to four cubes and imitate pencil strokes with a crayon. He may have six to ten words and may be able to carry out two directions. He may also have his toilet habits regulated in the daytime by this time.

GROWTH AND DEVELOPMENT—TWO YEARS TO NINE YEARS
2 Years of Age. By this time he can point to his eyes, nose, ears and *may* be toilet-trained during waking hours. He runs well without falling, can go up and down stairs alone, may kick a ball. He may use three-word sentences and may tell you when he needs to go to the bathroom. He may put on simple clothing himself and mimic certain play.

3 Years of Age. He may talk in short sentences, feed himself, and is generally toilet-trained. He alternates his feet going upstairs instead of putting one foot on a step and then bringing the other one to the same step. He may ride a tricycle. He can build a nine- or ten-cube tower. He can copy a circle and a cross. He can give his name and state whether he is a boy or a girl and usually obeys a few simple commands. He may feed himself well and be able to put on shoes and unbutton buttons. He may know some songs or rhymes and understand what it means to take turns.

4 Years of Age. He can walk downstairs alternating his feet. He can throw a ball and hop on one foot. He can draw the figure of a man with at least two parts to it, and copy a cross. He can count three objects and correctly point to them. He may name one or more colors accurately and obeys about five commands. He may be able to wash and dry his face; brush his teeth; tell the back from the front of clothes; lace his shoes and go on errands outside the home. He can play games and repeat four numbers.

5 Years of Age. He can speak in sentences of ten syllables; knows three or four colors; can name a nickel, a penny and a dime; can dress and undress without help; may ask the meaning of words; can draw a man with a body, head, and arms; can copy a triangle and circle; can count to ten; and can skip, alternating his feet.

6 Years of Age. He can tell his right from his left hand; can count to thirteen or thirty, can draw a man with neck, hands, and clothes; can add and subtract within 5; can repeat four numbers; can tie shoelaces; knows the difference between morning and night.

7 Years of Age. He knows the names of the days of the week and can repeat five numbers.

8 Years of Age. He can count backwards from 20.

9 Years of Age. By this age he can repeat the months, knows how to tell time, and can give change from a quarter.

GROWTH AND DEVELOPMENT—PHYSICAL

▶ **Height** The average birth length of a child is about 20 inches (50 cm.). In the first 6 months the child grows 1 inch a month; the second 6 months he grows one-half inch a month. At the end of the first year your child has increased his birth length by 50 per cent. By the fourth year he has doubled it. After that, the height increase is averaged at about 2 or 3 inches per year. By the thirteenth year, the birth length has tripled. From 1 to 7 years height increases 3 inches a year. From 8 to 15 years it increases 2 inches a year. From 16 to 20, it increases only 1 inch a year.

▶ **Weight** Birth—6 to 7½ to 9 pounds is the usual birth weight. The infant loses approximately 10 per cent of the birth weight during the first three or four days. This actually represents water loss, not weight. It is usually regained by the eighth or tenth day. First 6 months, gain is 6 to 8 ounces per week. Second 6 months, gain is 3 to 4 ounces per week. 5 months—birth weight doubles (14 pounds). 1 year—birth weight triples (21 pounds). 2½ years—birth weight quadruples (28 pounds). 5 years—weight at 1 year has doubled (42 pounds). 10 years—weight at 1 year has tripled (63 pounds). 13 to 14 years—weight at 1 year has quadrupled (84 pounds). Generally speaking, the average weight increase after the age of 2 is about 5 pounds per year until the ninth or tenth year. After this the weight curve decreases slowly. There is a rapid gain in weight during adolescence. A rough idea of weight during preschool and early school years can be gotten by using the following formula:

Age (in years) x 5, plus 18, equals weight in pounds.

▶ **Chest Measurements** The chest measurement at birth is about one half inch smaller than the head. At 1 year of age the chest is equal to, or slightly greater, than the head measurement, and after that it grows more rapidly. The circumference of the abdomen is generally about the same as that of the chest during the first year.

▶ **Heartrate** At birth, the heartrate is 140 beats per minute. At 6 months, 110 beats per minute; at 1 year, 100 beats per minute; at 3 to 4 years, 95 beats per minute; at 5 to 10 years, 90 beats per minute; at 10 to 15 years, 85 beats per minute; over 15 years, 75 to 80 beats per minute.

▶ **Breathing Rate** At birth, breathing rate is 40 per minute; at 6 months, 30 per minute; at 1 year, 28 per minute; at 3 to 4 years, 25 per minute; at 5 to 10 years, 24 per minute; at 10 to 15 years, 20 per minute; over 15, 12 to 18 per minute.

▶ **Speech** In the infant, all early sounds are impulsive and aimless. By two months of age they have generally become

cooing and gurgling sounds; at four months there are consonants followed by vowels; at eight months, certain syllables
and then "Mama" and "Dada." At eighteen months, words
may be accompanied by movements and gestures. At twenty-
four months, short sentences of three to four words, not necessarily grammatical, are heard.

▶ **Sight** When an infant is born, the pupils react to light but
light is generally avoided. At one month of age, the child can
follow a moving light. At seven weeks, he will close his lids
when a light is brought close. At two months, familiar objects
and faces are recognized. At four months, the infant reaches
for objects. At six to eight months, he transfers them from
one hand to the other. At twelve months, he may distinguish
colors in the following order: yellow, red, and then blue.

▶ **Taste, Touch, Smell** The sense of taste is present at birth,
but it is not known whether the child can differentiate sour,
salt, and bitter tastes. By two or three months, taste is acute
and the child can notice a change in the amounts of sugar or
other substances in his food. He begins to salivate at about
the third month. The lips and tongue of the infant are developed at birth. Localization of touch is developed by the
fifth month.

Sense of smell is present in the premature and normal-term
infant, but this develops slowly. It becomes more acute later
on. Most infants can smell milk.

▶ **Hearing** Hearing develops after the first few days of life,
but a deaf infant may show no signs of deafness for many
months. One of the first things noted in a deaf child would
be less-than-normal vocalization and not much laughter and
smiling. After about one month of age, the child can localize
and recognize where noises are coming from. By three months
of age he can recognize familiar voices, and after six months
may respond pleasurably to music. If the child is extremely
attentive visually, it may be a sign that hearing is not normal.
This should be quickly investigated, since a hearing defect
threatens a child's contact with his environment and may dis-
tort his entire behavior.

▶ **Sleep** Infants require a great deal of sleep during the first
few months of life—about eighteen to twenty hours per day
up until about six months of age, and by one year, fourteen
to sixteen hours. At two years the requirements are twelve to

fourteen hours, and at five years, ten to twelve hours. The need for sleep varies in children as it does in adults, and many children may give up naps earlier than others.

GROWTH AND DEVELOPMENT—BONES   The story of growth is basically the story of the bones. These are to the body as structural steel is to a building; both determine height and shape. Growth in the body is a most complex process and is more than a simple multiplication of cells. If one compares the face of the infant with that of the adult, it is easy to see the many changes in proportion that only *differential growth* can produce: the nose and the jaws must necessarily become larger, whereas the bones encasing the brain grow proportionately less prominent. Similar differential in growth occurs in the rest of the body, most notably, perhaps, in the lower extremities, in which relative shortness is found in infancy and early childhood.

Most growth that occurs around puberty seems to center in the region of the knees. Many complex factors operate in all this; one factor is the genes which will decree what the ultimate height and appearance of the individual will be. The various secretions of the endocrine glands are also necessary to set the stage properly for correct bone development. Thus, in hypothyroidism (underactive thyroid) there is a marked lag in skeletal growth. The administration of thyroid hormone produces a marked acceleration of growth; in fact, mildly hyperthyroid children tend to be taller. The vitamin D the child receives and the amount of calcium made available in the diet are also controlling factors in bone growth. It must be remembered also that there is a range of variability to growth. Some children lag behind others for no very definite reasons that can be ascertained. The gap is sometimes made up suddenly. A sex factor is also involved; girls may grow more rapidly than boys, and even exceed them in height, but with the onset of puberty and menstruation the female rate of growth decreases sharply; at the equivalent point, the boy may undergo a considerable and sustained spurt of growth.

▶ **Estimating Age by Bone Growth**   Many bones are formed from a cartilaginous model. Within the cartilage, centers for bone formation appear at stated times; these are known as centers of ossification. A good deal is known about the location and sequence of appearance of such centers. Thus, a few appropriately taken X-rays may enable the doctor to give an estimate of age. This figure is known as the bone age. If adverse influences have been operative (such as prolonged illness or poor nutrition) the bone age may lag behind the child's calendar age. Determination of bone age may be of value in such a situation as is presented by an adolescent of short stature; if bone age is less than calendar age, further growth and acceleration in height may be anticipated.

During early years, hands and wrists give excellent X-ray pictures for estimating bone age because of the numerous little bones present there and the sequence in which centers of ossification appear: at one year, there are two centers among the little bones of the wrist; at three, a third center appears (the triangularis); at four, a fourth center appears (the lunate); at five, two more appear (major multangulum and navicular); at six years a seventh center appears; and at ten years an eighth one. If, therefore, the wrist of a six-year-old fails to show either major or minor multangulum centers, or the navicular, although the lunate is present, bone age would be about four and a half—obviously well behind chronologic age. Similar useful data can be obtained later in childhood by X-raying such areas as the pelvis.

GROWTH AND DEVELOPMENT—HEAD The progress of growth is from the head down. Therefore, at birth, the head is relatively large, the trunk long, and the lower extremities relatively short. The arms are usually longer than the legs and the middle part of the body is about three-quarters of an inch above the umbilical cord. The extremities grow much more rapidly than the trunk, and the head grows the least. By approximately two years of age, the middle point of the body is slightly below the umbilicus. There are two "soft" spots on the head. The front one (fontanelle) is quadrangular in shape; it closes gradually as the cranial bones grow together. This soft spot represents the space between the cranial bones to permit expansion of the brain. It is generally closed by sixteen to eighteen months of age. The posterior fontanelle is closed at six to eight weeks. This is a triangular area at the back of the head.

► **Measurements of the Head** Circumference at birth is thirteen to fourteen inches. There is an increase of about one-half an inch a month, making a total of two inches (5 cm.) in the first four months of life. Another two-inch increase in the next eight months makes a total growth of over four inches (10 cm.) for the first year (to measure 17 to 18 inches). Second year growth is one inch (total 18 to 19 inches). From the end of the first year to the age of twenty, the head increases by only four inches in all, with growth between ages three to five years at the rate of one-half inch per year (19½ to 20½ inches), and one-half inch every five years thereafter until adult (20½ to 21½ inches).

GROWTH AND DEVELOPMENT—SPEECH DISORDERS

Development of speech in a child begins at birth and continues in regular and progressive developmental manner with increasing complexity for the rest of his life. This development of speech implies that the child's brain and central nervous system are normal. However, there are many reasons, both organic and psychological, which may impede, prevent, or disturb the development of proper communication, such as serious childhood illnesses, metabolic disorders, or malnutrition. Cleft palate and harelip, which result from embryonic defects, are organic causes of speech delay.

Many palsied children have difficulty in communication, ranging from complete inability to speak to disturbances in pronunciation and intelligibility.

Another organic cause of speech defect and inability to develop speech is called "congenital aphasia." This may result from an accident or illness before the speech process began. It is usually connected with brain damage.

Deafness will interfere with a child's learning to talk normally. This may cause him to appear mentally retarded.

The steps or phases of speech development are listed below:

1. *At birth,* and up until six to ten months, the child will gurgle, coo, babble, and make general vowel and consonant sounds.
2. *At ten months* most children will say "Mama" or "Dada."
3. *At eighteen months* the vocabulary contains about ten to twenty words and there may be small phrases.

194

4. *At thirty months* sentences involving a few words are usually developed. There may be some difficulty in articulating certain consonants such as *"s," "r" "l."* This slight difficulty in pronunciation frequently disappears. If it does not, speech therapy may be required.

5. *At thirty-six months* the child has all the mechanics of language at his command, and after this his speech development consists of vocabulary and grammar.

▶ **Speech Defects, Psychological Causes of** Speech, as communication of needs and desires, is a primary need. Its frustration always has consequences. These may be reactions of aggression, hostility, and resentment. Since such emotions are not rewarding ones, they produce secondary developments of feelings of discouragement, inferiority, shame, and insecurity. A speech defect may result from a poor relationship of the child with his parents or may impair the relationship. Speech defects often have long-range and serious lifetime consequences. They may reduce his earning power by limiting his ability to work; alter his personality by undermining his self-esteem and personal adjustment; interfere with personal relationships and his general ability to communicate.

Children who have been given psychological tests to determine what factors were important in their poor speech development showed that *lack of a feeling of achievement, a feeling of anxiety and insecurity coupled with hostility* and *no hope of escape* were factors involved in their difficulties. Sometimes these findings may be secondary, as a *result* of an organic speech defect which causes interpersonal difficulties between the child and his parents. Some children are punished for not speaking properly. They are scolded, slapped, given whippings, and otherwise rigidly disciplined. Many of these children withdraw and respond with silence. Some of them develop stammering and stuttering. Any child who does not have understandable speech by the age of three years should certainly have a complete physical and psychological evaluation.

GROWTH AND DEVELOPMENT—PUBERTY Puberty
begins earlier in girls than in boys. It may start at eleven or twelve in girls, at thirteen to fifteen in boys. It is marked by extra growth in height and weight, and the development of

secondary sexual characteristics—menstruation, breast and pubic hair development in girls, and voice change and development of genital hair in boys. Emotionally, puberty is a stage between the giving up of childhood and its dependence on the parents, and the development of adolescence and independence. It is usually marked by a stormy course of emotional swings between rebellion and compliance. It marks the insurgence of sexual feelings and the desire to experiment. It is a period where the balance between freedom and license may be difficult to impose. If a youngster has had a good and stable relationship with his parents all of his life, he can usually emerge from adolescence with very little difficulty. Children who have had a disturbed emotional development become more disturbed with the pressures of puberty. Puberty is a period when there is still a need for parental guidance, but also a recognition that it is necessary to separate from the parents and become an independent, mature, functioning adult able to carry on one's own life. Parents often do not recognize this need and may prolong the period of dependence because of their own unsatisfied emotional needs.

Serious behavior disorders and delinquencies which occur at this time of the child's life usually require professional psychiatric help. The parents may also require treatment.

A condition that often disturbs parents of boys reaching puberty is nocturnal emission (wet dreams). Nocturnal emissions are experienced by adolescent boys as an emission of seminal fluid during the night when they are asleep. They awaken to find that the bedclothes are wet. These emissions are unconsciously produced, frequently due to the emerging sexual dreams and fantasies of this age. They are very common and harmless and should not be taken seriously. They are considered normal phenomena.

HEADACHE   The number of causes of headache are legion. Some of the more common ones include psychologic tension, inadequate sleep, respiratory and other viral illnesses, hangovers, menstruation, high blood pressure, eye strain, and various digestive disorders (including in some cases constipation). More serious but fortunately rare causes of headache will include certain inflammations of the brain, such as meningitis, brain tumors, and suppurative infections of the skull.

Some headaches are descriptively classified as simple head-ache (not due to any significant underlying causes), vascular headache (one with a throbbing quality), and tension headache which arises from tightening-up of the muscles at the back of the head and in the scalp. Migraine, also known as "sick head-ache," is a vascular headache which often starts with visual difficulties, is generally one-sided, and terminates with nausea and vomiting. It runs in families and occurs most often in tense, perfectionistic people with high standards and higher-than-average intelligence. Migraine is one of the few head-aches with a specifically reversible cause: a vasoconstrictive drug known as ergotamine when taken early in the attack may successfully reverse it. In many instances it is not possible to identify a special cause for headache.

Treatment. Treatment is therefore directed against the symp-tom—that is, the pain—and consists of various pain-killing medications starting with such drugs as aspirin and working upwards to drugs such as Darvon®, codeine and its derivatives, and even some of the narcotics. Most patients who have re-peated headaches find it worthwhile to experiment with several medications to see which is most effective. Sometimes com-binations of aspirin with small doses of benzedrine (Edrisal®, Daprisal®) may help some vascular headaches—particularly if one's blood pressure tends to be on the low-normal or low side. Another product found to help many chronic headache suffer-ers at the Montefiore Hospital Headache Clinic is Fiorinal®. Relief can sometimes be gotten by as simple a device as an icebag, or by taking aspirin and a short nap. Chronic or re-peated headache can be the subject of elaborate investigation including skull X-rays, brain-wave patterns, and detailed neuro-logical examination. Even these elaborate or refined techniques may fail to uncover an underlying disease process. The head-ache victim may well furnish meaningful clues by close observa-tions of the past pattern of his headaches, and report the data he secures to the doctor.

HEARTBURN   Heartburn is a term used for a burning sensation generally felt high in the upper central abdomen. It is experienced by many people after eating spicy, rich, greasy, or fried foods or after they have taken too much coffee or alco-hol. It is a common complaint during pregnancy, when it is due to various functional changes in the behavior of the digestive tract. Heartburn is probably not due to "excess acidity," but neutralizing stomach acids will help heartburn as well as other digestive complaints.

Treatment. Many over-the-counter remedies are sold for heartburn but they often contain bicarbonate of soda, too much of which is particularly undesirable during pregnancy. A milk-of-magnesia tablet is probably preferable for the pregnant woman and there are other alkalinizers—Amphogel®, Gelusil®, Maalox®, Riopan®, Titralac®, etc.—free of bicarbonate of soda. Many come in either liquid or tablet form, and whichever is easier to take can be used. Generally, one or two tablets or a teaspoonful or two of these medications will give some relief. It may be necessary to repeat the dose within an hour or two. Repeated or frequent heartburn may require consultation with a doctor. Occasionally further investigations, including stomach X-rays, may be in order if a ready explanation is not at hand. (See also HERNIA, HIATUS.)

HEART DISEASE, CONGENITAL   The symptoms of congenital heart disease may be noted from time of birth. A murmur may be heard immediately or within a few months after birth. Certain symptoms such as a bluish tinge to the skin, difficulty in breathing, and poor growth and development may be seen early. There is usually no history of rheumatic heart disease.

Congenital heart disease is divided into two main classifications: those which cause bluish discoloration of the skin (cyanotic) and those which do not (acyanotic). There are also "late cyanotic" ones. In the latter cases the blue color does not develop until the child is older.

In cyanotic congenital heart disease there is an abnormal communication between the pulmonic and systemic circulations. Fresh blood from the lungs mixes with bluish blood from the returned systemic circulation, and the result is a mixture which causes the bluish discoloration of the skin.

In the acyanotic group there is no abnormal communication between the left and right side, therefore no mixture of blood and no bluish discoloration. However, other conditions which cause abnormalities may give a very poor prognosis for life and health.

In the late cyanotic groups, there is an arterial venous shunt (communication between the right and left sides of the heart, or between the systemic and pulmonic circulation). Normally, the pressure on the left side of the heart is higher than that of the right. However, if there is a complication in which the pressure on the right side is raised above that on the left, there will be a reversal of blood flow, the shunt will become venous to arterial, and cyanosis will develop. This may be a late finding in certain forms of heart abnormalities.

The prognosis for children with certain forms of congenital heart disease has been improved tremendously by the modern advances of open heart surgery. Even for children who have destructive valvular lesions due to rheumatic heart disease, such as mitral stenosis and other valvular insufficiencies, the prognosis is also much better due to new surgical techniques. There is now a pulmonary-circulation machine which continuously oxygenates the blood during heart surgery.

HEAT REACTIONS   Reactions to excessive heat may take several forms. *Heat exhaustion* occurs most often during spells of hot, humid weather. The person will complain of faintness, dizziness, weakness. The skin will be moist but not hot. Occasionally there will be nausea and muscular or abdominal cramps. The following steps should be followed for heat exhaustion: (1) Have the person stretch out in as cool and open a spot as is available. (2) Give small frequent sips of cold drinks, such as fruit juices, to which extra salt has been added. If there has been a good deal of perspiration, salt tablets can be given. Stimulants such as coffee or tea, iced or otherwise, may also be given. The face and extremities may be rubbed down with cold cloths.

Heat stroke is most often seen after considerable exposure to the sun, at the beach or in the country. In heat stroke the body's temperature-regulating mechanism goes astray, and the victim is obviously very hot to the touch. In fact, temperatures ranging up to 106 degrees have occurred in heat stroke. The skin is hot and dry, the pulse rapid and strong. Weakness and headache are the usual complaints.

Treatment. The victim should be helped out of the sun into as cool a spot as possible. Measures designed to reduce the body temperature should be instituted promptly. These may range from dousing the person with cold water to applications of ice to various parts of the body. Alcohol may be freely applied, as it too may efficiently lower body temperature. Cold applications should be continued if the patient is transported to a hospital.

HEMORRHOIDS   Hemorrhoids are small distended veins in the region of the anus or rectal opening. The ones just inside the opening are covered by the lining of the anus and are called internal hemorrhoids; those exterior to this are covered by skin and are called external hemorrhoids. Anything that raises the pressure within the veins of the rectal region may bring on or aggravate hemorrhoids. Pregnancy is one of the most common aggravating factors, as are also chronic constipation and straining at stool.

Many individuals have one or two hemorrhoids without being aware of them, and certainly such asymptomatic hemorrhoids need cause no concern. Sometimes, however, hemorrhoids appear in clusters like small grapes and are readily felt externally when wiping after a movement. They become quite painful, until sitting is uncomfortable or impossible. Such pain is often brought on by a clotting within the hemorrhoid—a thrombosed hemorrhoid. Occasionally, because of impaired blood supply to the skin over the hemorrhoid, an ulcer may form with severe pain resulting.

Hemorrhoids often present a problem of acute or emergency nature and certain first aid measures may be useful: (1) Cold compresses of plain water or of half water, half witch hazel may provide relief. (2) Hot sitz baths may also relieve the pain of hemorrhoids and help stop bleeding. A sitz bath is prepared by drawing four to six inches of hot water in the tub and sitting in it. (3) Sometimes hemorrhoids will produce annoying oozing or staining for which a sanitary napkin applied to the rectum may be useful. (4) During the painful stage of hemorrhoids a rubber ring, or the adjustment of two small pillows so that the buttocks are supported without pressure against the anal region, may make life more tolerable.

The doctor may, after a preliminary anesthetic to the area, cut into a thrombosed hemorrhoid and evacuate the clot; this will often relieve the pain or at least diminish it considerably. Generally, a hot sitz bath is prescribed after this procedure.

For multiple hemorrhoids which are chronic and annoying, or which bleed frequently, surgical removal is generally curative. Considerable relief may be secured by the local application of hemorrhoid ointment, or the insertion into the anus of special suppositories containing anesthetics and certain healing agents. (See also SUPPOSITORIES.)

HEPATITIS   Hepatitis refers to a variety of inflammations of the liver, including those produced by viruses, amoebas, and even various drugs. Unless otherwise qualified, however, it generally refers to a virus-produced condition, *viral hepatitis* (for which the synonyms are "infectious hepatitis" and also "serum hepatitis"). Viral hepatitis seems to be on the increase in recent years. The early symptoms may be grippe-like, with chilly feelings, headache, fever, and a loss of appetite. At about the same time it may be noted that the urine is darker than usual. This is brought about by an excess of bile pigments in the blood, which spill over into the urine. In jaundiced cases, there is a yellow tint to the skin and whites of the eyes. This usually deepens so that over the course of the next week or two deep yellow staining may become obvious. The stools are generally lighter than normal. The jaundice is produced because the damaged liver cells can no longer perform their proper functions, one of which is to transfer bile pigments out of the bloodstream and into the intestines. Even mild cases seldom clear in less than three to four weeks, and a six- to eight-week period of illness is by no means uncommon. Complete recovery is the rule, although in a small minority the condition may become chronic.

Viral hepatitis is a contagious disease, although it is not common to see more than one case in a household. Probably most cases are the result of contamination of food by an infected person who may not have symptoms. In fact, most cases of this disease do not produce obvious jaundice and are referred to as anicteric (non-jaundice) cases. Hence many adults without a history of jaundice have, in fact, had the disease and are immune.

A disease quite indistinguishable from naturally occurring hepatitis can be transmitted by blood transfusion and blood products; it is therefore known as *serum hepatitis*. It may come on a month or more after receiving a blood transfusion which contained the virus.

Treatment. The disease is customarily treated by rest, which is not necessarily strict bed rest, a high-carbohydrate diet (high also in proteins, if the patient can tolerate them), and in a few instances steroid drugs may be employed. It is customary to give an injection of gamma globulin to household contacts, and it has been demonstrated in institutional outbreaks that gamma globulin injections can stop an epidemic. Some recent work indicates that serum hepatitis may also be reduced in intensity, if not prevented, by giving one large dose of gamma globulin at the time of the transfusion and another approximately one month later.

HERNIA A hernia is an abnormal protrusion of a bodily organ into a canal or opening. The opening may be one normally present in the body but abnormally enlarged, or it may be an opening artificially created—as, for example, after surgery. Most common hernias are in close relation to the abdominal cavity and frequently contain a portion of the digestive tract. One common form of hernia seen in infants, and occasionally in adults, occurs at the "belly button" (umbilicus) and is called an *umbilical hernia.* In infants it is often temporary and requires only adhesive-taping.

The inguinal canal in males is a frequent site for *inguinal hernia.* This is the oblique canal which penetrates the abdominal musculature, and through which runs the spermatic cord that sends sperm up from the testicles. Normally, the fibrous connective tissue and muscle defining the inguinal canal snugly enclose the spermatic cord and resist any encroachment from adjacent structures. Occasionally, perhaps because of a slight defect in construction of the canal or from excessive intra-abdominal pressure, a "knuckle" of intestine may work its way into the aperture. As time goes by the aperture tends to widen, hence hernias tend to grow larger. In a full-fledged inguinal hernia, a fair-sized loop of bowel may have worked its way down into the scrotum. Generally it can be tucked back into the abdomen and is referred to as a *reducible* hernia.

Apart from being a nuisance, the hernia may present no threat; many individuals get along without paying much attention to them. The chief threat may not arise for years, if at all—this threat being a twisting or swelling within the herniated bowel loop following which it can no longer be replaced. This is known as an *incarcerated* hernia. Incarceration may present all the features of an intestinal obstruction; in addition, the bowel may become acutely inflamed because its own blood supply can be cut off. This produces a surgical emergency requiring active intervention.

For uncomplicated hernia, belts with padding (trusses) may be arranged so as to keep the hernia tucked within the abdominal cavity. But individuals who wear these trusses often complain of some discomfort from the pressure they exert. Another drawback is that the truss has to be worn constantly. To avoid both the risks and discomfort of hernia, surgical repair is often advised. The procedure is known as a herniorrhaphy. Inguinal hernias also occur in women, though to a lesser extent than in men. Relatively more common in women are hernias which present in the upper portion of the thigh just beneath the abdominal crease. They are called *femoral hernias* and have much the same significance as does an inguinal hernia.

HERNIA, HIATUS   The food-pipe (esophagus) is a long, slender, muscular tube which runs from the back of the throat down to the stomach. Just before it opens into the stomach it penetrates the diaphragm through a special opening known as the hiatus. Several factors may produce widening of the hiatus, which in turn leads to the appearance of a portion of stomach above the level of the diaphragm. It may take a special maneuver to reveal the widening, since the stomach is not always herniated through the opening.

Most cases of hiatus hernia cause no distress or discomfort. They may be discovered as an incidental finding in an X-ray study. However, a hiatus hernia may lead to symptoms of pressure—often interpreted as a heart pain—and palpitations or cardiac irregularities. Upper-abdominal discomfort is sometimes also felt in the back, with associated symptoms such as burping and belching. Attacks may be intermittent and are sometimes relieved by shifting from the lying to the standing position. There is a tendency to ascribe too many symptoms to a really innocent hiatus hernia.

Many common forms of indigestion and such everyday symptoms as heartburn or burping occur in individuals without hiatus hernia. In the few cases where it is clear that a hiatus hernia is producing frequent symptoms or contributing to chronic anemia, an operation may be advised. This consists basically of "taking tucks" into the widened hiatus and thereby narrowing the opening. Since no organ needs to be cut into in this repair, the operative procedure generally poses no particular difficulty.

Treatment. Medical treatment of hiatus hernia resembles that used for the treatment of peptic ulcer. Alkalinizers, to be taken at frequent intervals throughout the day, may be prescribed. Since overdistention of the stomach should be avoided, the patient with hiatus hernia will do better to eat small frequent meals rather than a few large ones. In a few instances, raising the head of the bed may prevent night attacks; weight reduction may also be quite helpful.

HOME CARE DURING ILLNESS

▶ **Caring For a Sick Child** The following are a few important considerations to keep in mind when taking care of a sick child:

1. Do not give any medicine, patent or otherwise, except perhaps aspirin, unless you have consulted your doctor.

2. Do not follow the recommendations of your neighbor who gave her child a particular medicine. Chances are her child had a totally different illness although the symptoms may have seemed similar.

3. Do not give enemas without the consent or advice of your doctor. *You* may think the child's bellyache is merely constipation or "something he ate." It may really be acute appendicitis. It is extremely dangerous to introduce water under pressure when the appendix is inflamed, since this may cause the appendix to rupture.

4. Do not give laxatives routinely to "clean a child out." This is an unnecessary habit and is potentially harmful. The child who has difficulty passing stools should have medical advice and investigation to determine the reason for this.

5. Severe and prolonged illnesses in children create special problems. Diseases such as tuberculosis, rheumatic fever, or paralytic polio create secondary psychological dependency problems in the child and often produce great anxiety in the parents. As a result, the child may become a chronic invalid,

mentally as well as physically. It is important to give these children as much psychological freedom as possible so that their physical illness does not permanently warp their personalities. It is much safer not to discuss the child's illness, length of illness, future, etc., in his presence either with the doctor or with relatives. Nor should it be discussed with his playmates. It may cause misunderstandings and result in severe permanent psychological damage. A child can be kept busy, active, and interested in various forms of occupational therapy while he is ill, so that he can make progress in other areas and not have time to brood about his condition.

▶ **Feeding a Sick Child** Most sick children have no appetite for solid foods. The best thing to do is to nourish them with some form of fruit or fruit juices, liquids, such as bouillon, weak tea, clear soup, sodas, milk, and even ice cream. A mashed banana may be given in orange juice, or other fresh fruit mashed in fruit juice. This provides glucose (sugar) and fluid. Other foods which are both good and easy to take are soft things such as Jello, custard, rice pudding, mashed potatoes, or any easy-to-swallow food. If a child continues to vomit there is medicine which can be given to stop the vomiting. For children who have to maintain a high nutrition and calorie intake, there are prepared food supplements which can be bought. They are effective in providing all the nourishment (calories, protein, fat, and carbohydrates) which a growing child requires, in a liquid form.

▶ **Giving Medicine** Some children will take any medicine which is offered to them. Others will take it providing it does not taste very bad. But there are some who are extremely particular and will refuse anything that tastes strange. In such cases it is possible to get medication into these children, sometimes a drop at a time, if it can be mixed with something pleasant-tasting which the child already likes. It may be mixed, drop-by-drop, with one or two ounces of cherry soda, ice cream, applesauce, or jam. Sometimes it can be placed in rice pudding, tapioca, or malted milks. Most modern medications are so pleasant (or tasteless) that they can be mixed into almost any pleasant food. For children who absolutely refuse anything by mouth, many medications can be administered by injection; others can be administered rectally. Aspirin is available in the form of rectal suppositories, and so are other pain-killing drugs. Your physician will advise you whether this is necessary.

► **How to Give an Enema** You will need an enema bag with tubing and an enema tip; a bedpan, newspaper, some toilet paper, vaseline or cold cream, and a small rubber sheet or oilcloth. There are some prepared enemas which can be bought in the drugstore in a prepared plastic bottle with a nozzle. After being lubricated, the appropriately sized nozzle is simply inserted into the child's rectum and the material in the bottle is squeezed into the rectal area. In a homemade enema, the water should be lukewarm and, generally, mild soapsuds used. The water is placed in the enema bag with the soapsuds and shaken up a bit. The bedclothes are turned back and an oilcloth or protective toweling is placed under the child. The bag is hung low enough so that the water goes into the rectum very slowly. The enema solution should be retained by the patient for two to five minutes if possible. Then the child may be placed on the bedpan or the toilet and the contents expelled. You always wash your own hands and the patient's hands after enemas. The enema bag should be cleansed thoroughly after use; the enema bone may be sterilized by boiling for five minutes.

Another type of enema for a very constipated stool is the oil-retention enema. Two to four ounces of mineral oil are inserted into the rectum and held there for five to ten minutes so that the stool may be softened. Then it is expelled.

► **Setting up the Sick Room** The behavior of a child who is sick will depend directly upon how severe his illness is. With an extremely high fever—103° or 104°F.—he will not be anxious to play. He is *really* sick: he may be cranky, irritable, fussy or want to sleep most of the time, in which case it is best to let him do so. Many children who are sick cannot concentrate on games, television, or other activities which normally interest them. However, a child who is bedridden but not very toxic requires distraction and things to play with because he becomes annoyed and bored at being confined to bed. There are things which may make a child more comfortable and will divert him (and permit you to do less running around). If he has the following items near his bedside it will be much easier to keep him happy and occupied: Drinking water or soda with ice cubes, a glass, a spoon, and tissues are essentials; also a bag for waste material pinned to the mattress or a small wastebasket placed by the bed. A large shopping bag can contain most of his toys, crayons, paint books, magazines, or other handicraft material. A small radio, or possibly a television set which is not too far from the foot of the bed so that he can manipulate the dials, is a welcome diversion.

Materials which encourage creative interest and skills are excellent diversions for a sick child. Coloring paper, pencils, art handicraft supplies, knitting, embroidery and sewing things are interesting. Tropical fish, a bird or other pets may create diversion. Hobbies such as stamp-collecting, shell-collecting, making a scrapbook, or keeping a diary can be encouraged at this time. Modeling with clay is also very useful. If a child has to be kept in bed, he may be permitted to lie in the living room on the couch rather than in bed. This allows him to partake in the general family life rather than feeling isolated.

The most important thing in caring for a sick child is not to permit him to become so accustomed to overwhelming attention that when he gets well his personality will again become directed to absorbing all this attention toward himself. It is important not to hover over him to the point where he becomes helpless and dependent. When he is again well, he should be treated without the concern and anxiety you naturally felt when he was ill.

▶ **Recognizing Illness in Children up to Two Years of Age**

How do you know when a child who cannot speak is ill? By the time your child is one or two years old, you know him pretty well. You know his moods, his general behavior, and whether he is cheerful, contented, happy, playful. You know when he is wet, when he wishes to be picked up, when he's hungry, tired, or needs a nap. If your child is behaving in a manner which is not up to his usual standard, he may be coming down with some illness. It is wise to check his temperature at this time. If he is extremely irritable, cranky, fussy, refuses to eat, doesn't play with his toys, seems listless, apathetic, sleeps a lot, etc., these may be signs of illness. Some mothers think they can tell a child's temperature by feeling his forehead. This is usually not accurate since a low-grade temperature of 100°F. or so is not always felt on touching the skin. If the temperature is over 100°, one can assume that an illness is developing. It is wise to check the temperature again within an hour or so. Many children with temperatures of 103° or 104°F. appear perfectly normal, cheerful, active, and show no signs of illness, whereas others with only slight temperatures may show listlessness and a lack of playful activity. (See also FEVER.)

▶ **Preparing Children for Hospital** Children who are ill and must undergo hospitalization or surgery should be prepared for it beforehand if their age permits. Most children of four, five, and up can understand what you tell them. These children should be informed (depending on their age level and degree of understanding) in a calm, matter-of-fact manner as to what they are to expect. Fear and anxiety should be minimized. If they are left alone in a hospital where painful things are done to them in a strange atmosphere without any explanation, they may become very frightened and traumatized. Sudden experiences with anesthesia are often interpreted by the child as being "smothered." This, too, can have traumatic psychological effects. A good general rule is to realize that it is not wise to lie to children about their future experiences in any area. It may be necessary to give explanations which are not completely accurate and descriptive, but adequate at least to the level of their own understanding. If children find that you lie to them, trick them and disappoint them often, they will lose confidence in you and never believe anything you say. This will shake their belief and trust in people in general and make them uncertain of themselves and their experiences.

Failure to prepare children for painful experiences often results in behavior disturbances. They start having nightmares, phobias, nervousness, wakefulness, and sometimes permanent impairment of the personality may result from shock. Modern practice today is to permit the parents to be in the same room with the child following an operation or, whenever possible, at least to be present when the child emerges from anesthesia and is out of danger.

With the use of modern antibiotics, only acute emergencies, accidents, severe croup, convulsions, meningitis, appendicitis, poisonings, and elective surgery require hospitalization. Most pneumonia can be treated at home providing there are no complications. Even tuberculosis is often treated at home. Diseases for which hospitalization is required have been enormously reduced in number in the past twenty years. Most doctors will attempt to take care of a child at home if at all possible.

HORMONES AND GLANDS   The hormones are "chemical messengers" produced by glands located in various parts of the body. One feature they share in common is that the secretion is poured directly into the bloodstream and affects the function of an organ or organs in a distant location. (The organ affected is sometimes referred to as the "target organ.") The glands are sometimes collectively termed the endocrines. Some of the more important glands and hormones are described below:

1. *Pituitary.* This tiny gland at the base of the brain has a dominant role because many of its target organs are other endocrine glands. The pituitary secretes gonadotropic hormones which stimulate the ovary and testicle to secrete the sex hormones. Other pituitary hormones are *ACTH,* which stimulates the adrenal gland to secrete hydrocortisone and related chemicals; the mammotropic hormone, which stimulates the breast to produce milk and becomes particularly operative toward the end of pregnancy, and the somatotropic hormone, which stimulates growth. Somatotropic hormone is in short supply but has been shown experimentally to increase the growth of human dwarfs.

2. *Sex hormones.* These include testosterone in the male, which is secreted by the testicles, and in the female, estrogen and progesterone secreted by the ovaries. Small amounts of sex hormones are also secreted by the adrenals in both sexes.

3. *Adrenal.* This pair of glands produces a complex group of hormones which regulate such basic processes as the formation of fats and sugars, the secretion of urine, and bodily responses to inflammation.

4. *Thyroid.* Controlled by a pituitary factor known as TSH (thyroid stimulating hormone), the thyroid gland in turn produces a hormone, thyroxin, which stimulates all processes in all cells of the body.

5. *Insulin.* This is a hormone (produced by the pancreas) which regulates the level of the blood sugar and controls the rate at which the blood sugar enters cells.

6. *Miscellaneous other hormones include:* Secretin, a digestive tract hormone which stimulates the pancreas; cholecysto-

209

kinin, a similar hormone, which stimulates the gallbladder to contract; ADH, a hormone produced by the posterior part of the pituitary gland, which regulates urine formation, and oxytocin, another posterior pituitary substance, which produces contractions of the uterus.

▶ **Endocrine Diseases** The thyroid, pituitary, pineal, adrenal, parathyroid, ovary, testes, and pancreas are endocrine glands, or glands of internal secretion. They secrete chemicals (called hormones) which have a complex functional interrelationship in both health and disease.

During the first few weeks of life there may be carry-over effects of the mother's hormones, producing various conditions in the infant, such as swollen breasts, vaginal discharge, and uterine bleeding. They may cause secretion of milk in the breasts of both male and female infants. The thyroid and pituitary glands are usually well-developed at birth.

Hypoparathyroidism (under-development of parathyroid gland) may cause symptoms of tetany in the newborn, i.e., crowing breathing, generalized convulsions, and carpopedal spasm (in which the wrist is flexed, the hand bent back, and the thumb is in the cupped palm). There is a decrease in the amounts of ionized calcium in the blood, causing hyperirritability of the neuromuscular system. There may be other causes of tetany, but an under-developed parathyroid gland is most common.

Hypothyroidism may be present at birth or acquired later. It is also called cretinism. The absence or lack of thyroid gland in non-goitrous geographic areas causes the "occasional" form of cretinism. In goitrous areas the condition is due to deficiency of thyroid hormone secretion (endemic form).

Cretinism is a condition of mental retardation due to lack of thyroid hormone, associated with the following signs: coarse brittle hair, cool thick skin, stunted height, delayed teething, large tongue, infantile face and body proportions, pot-belly with poor muscle tone, and intolerance to cold. Cretinous children show physical, mental, and emotional retardation. There are characteristic laboratory blood findings and X-ray findings. Usually the protein-bound serum-iodine level is low, testing with radioactive iodine showing low or absent levels.

The treatment of cretinism is substitution therapy with thyroid hormone. Naturally, the earlier these children are diagnosed and treated, the better the prognosis.

Hyperthyroidism is a condition of excess secretion of thyroid hormone due to a nodule (toxic adenoma) or Graves' disease (toxic goiter). The latter, more common in younger persons, is due to overstimulation of the thyroid gland by the pituitary. These patients show hyperactivity, nervousness, tremors, rapid heart rate, high blood pressure, bulging eyes (exophthalmos), loss of weight with accelerated growth in children, and emotional instability. Blood tests of protein-bound iodine in the serum and uptake of radioactive iodine show increased levels. The basic metabolic rate is increased.

Treatment of hyperthyroidism is directed towards suppressing the effect of the overactive thyroid gland with medicine. If the symptoms of hyperthyroidism do not subside on medical management, surgical removal of the thyroid gland may be necessary.

HYSTERECTOMY   Surgical removal of the uterus (womb) is the operation referred to as a hysterectomy. In some instances the cervix may be left in, the operation then being termed a supracervical hysterectomy. When the cervix too is removed, the procedure is referred to as a complete hysterectomy. Still another variant is a panhysterectomy, in which the tubes and ovaries are also removed (pan = all).

The most common cause of hysterectomy is the growth of the benign tumors known as fibroids. A uterus enlarged because of fibroids may produce uncomfortable pressure symptoms and interference with the function of nearby organs, most often the bladder. Very heavy and prolonged menstrual periods or other forms of frequent and recurrent uterine bleeding, when not controllable by other measures, may necessitate a hysterectomy. Cancer of the uterus is often treated in this way, sometimes after a preliminary period of irradiation. Rather rarely, some severe and life-threatening infections of the uterus may also lead to hysterectomy.

When the ovaries are removed in a premenopausal woman, a surgical menopause follows. Like the naturally occurring menopause, it too may be marked by flushes and sweats, and these may sometimes be severe. It too may require the use

211

of hormones for a variable period of time. The tides of medical opinion have changed over the years as to whether or not it is wise to remove the ovaries at the time of hysterectomy.

One of the arguments for a panhysterectomy is that since tumor formation is by no means rare in the ovaries, their removal at the time of the hysterectomy can be regarded as justifiable prophylaxis. A decisive factor may be age: a surgeon would certainly feel less hesitant about removing the ovaries of a woman in her mid-forties, presumably approaching the menopause anyway. Fortunately, most of the mandatory reasons for doing hysterectomies are found in women in the older age group. In most instances these women have had their families so that the loss of the uterus has far less impact on them. A hysterectomy need in no way impair a woman's sexual life thereafter.

IMMUNIZATION OF YOUR CHILD   There are many diseases today which your child will never get if he is immunized against them. In previous years thousands of children used to die, during epidemics, of diseases which can now be prevented. It is therefore important and necessary for you to give your child all the injections which have been developed to protect him. Epidemics still can and do break out, but if this occurs your child will be protected. You can get in touch with your physician to arrange for this vital protection.

Long-term immunity can be given against smallpox, tuberculosis, polio, tetanus, whooping cough, diphtheria, and measles. If you are traveling outside the United States, especially to a tropical area, there are other diseases against which your child can be protected, such as typhoid-paratyphoid fever, yellow fever, cholera, typhus, and a few other very specialized diseases. Lifelong immunity cannot really be given against any disease by a single inoculation; therefore it is necessary at various ages to reinforce first injections with booster shots of the immunizing substance.

Temporary immunity can often be given a child against a disease to which he has been exposed before being inoculated against it. For example, if your child has been exposed to measles before he has received the measles vaccine, let your doctor know at once. The doctor will treat him with gamma globulin, which produces temporary immunity and will make the attack milder.

The ideal time for a child to start having his injections is about two to three months after birth. Always contact your physician during an epidemic, even if your child has received immunization; additional protection may be received in the form of booster doses. It is important to keep a record of the dates of your child's immunizations, so that you will know what he has been given and when it is time for booster injections. This record will be required almost every year that he registers in school, so keep it some place where you will have it readily available. A sample *Immunization Record* form appears on the next page.

IMMUNIZATION RECORD FOR _____
(Your Child's Name)

(Your doctor may follow a slightly different schedule)

	Recommended age	Date given
First Year		
DPT*	1½ to 2 months	_____
	3 months	_____
	5 months	_____
Polio vaccine	5-8 months	_____
Measles vaccine	6-12 months	_____
Smallpox vaccine	Before 12 months	_____
Second Year		
Give any injections not started or completed in first year.		
Additional injection of DPT.	12-18 months	_____
Polio and measles vaccine may be recommended by your doctor.		
Before Going to School		
DPT and polio vaccine	4 years	_____
Smallpox vaccine	5-6 years	_____
Thereafter		
Booster doses of DT (whooping cough no longer needed) and polio vaccine.	At intervals recommended by your doctor.	_____
Smallpox vaccine every 5 years, before the child leaves the United States or if there is an epidemic.		

*DPT stands for diphtheria, pertussis (whooping cough), and tetanus.

214

INFANT AND CHILDHOOD DISORDERS

▶ **Intussusception** Intussusception is an acquired form of intestinal obstruction and occurs mostly in young male children. A portion of the lower intestine turns inside of itself and blocks the linings and passage of food. It causes severe colicky pain, fever, and typical currant-jelly bowel movements. This represents some passage of blood in the stools. A sausage-shaped mass may sometimes be felt in the abdomen.

This condition requires immediate attention. The longer one delays diagnosis, the more difficult it is to treat. If it exists for more than twelve hours, strangulation of the bowel and gangrene may occur. The intussusception may sometimes reduce itself without treatment and not require surgery.

▶ **Infantile Tetany (Spasmophilia)** This is a neuromuscular hyperexcitability produced by inadequate amounts of ionized calcium in the blood. It is commonly associated with rickets, and is most frequently seen in male children during the first two years of life. A typical sign is "carpopedal spasm," in which the wrist is flexed, with the fingers extended and the hand abducted (turned), with the thumb in the cupped palm. Convulsions and crowing sounds when breathing in may occur. A blood test will show low calcium. The treatment is replacement therapy with intravenous or oral calcium.

▶ **Cleft Palate (Harelip)** During the fifth and eighth weeks in the developing embryo, the maxillary and premaxillary palatal processes fuse. A failure in fusion may result in either cleft lip or cleft palate, or both. The exact cause is unknown, but any abnormal influence occurring at a critical developmental level will cause defects in the developing embryo. This disorder is more frequent in males, and occurs in one in 800 births. Due to the space created, it may cause immediate feeding problems. Special methods of nursing may be required for these children. Most of these lesions are correctable with plastic surgery. This is performed at optimum growth periods, when all the available tissue may be used.

▶ **Thrush** This is an acute, sub-acute, or chronic infection caused by a yeastlike fungus called *monilia*. It may cause infections in any area of the body, but the most common type observed in newborn infants involves the mucous membranes of the mouth. Mouth thrush is characterized by white plaques on the tongue, cheek lining, and throat. It may be very painful and cause feeding difficulties.

Diagnosis can usually be made by simple observation or by culturing the fungus. *Candida albicans* usually causes these infections. The antibiotic Mycostatin is effective in clearing the lesions. Painting the mouth with aqueous gentian violet solution is also effective.

INFANT FEEDING

▶ **Breast-feeding** Breast-feeding of infants is generally to be encouraged because mother's milk is a truly natural source of food. It is more digestible than prepared milks and causes few feeding difficulties. The breasts should be emptied by the nursing child. The mother's diet should be adequate in nutritious food, vitamins, calories, and minerals. A relaxed attitude and freedom from tension and irritation are important factors in insuring an adequate breast-milk supply. Emptying the breasts is the best stimulus to refilling them. If breast-feeding is not possible, or if it is not desired, formula feeding is widely and generally accepted as an excellent substitute. If breast-feeding is only partially satisfactory, supplementary feedings with formula may be added. At four to six months, the infant can be weaned by the gradual substitution of formula feedings for breast-feeding.

The total daily fluid requirements for infants are approximately 2½ ounces per pound of body weight per day. Evaporated milk provides 40 calories to the ounce. Cow's or breast milk provides 20 calories per ounce. Sugar (2 tablespoons) equals 120 calories per ounce, corn syrup, 120 calories per 2 tablespoons. Dextri-maltose equals 120 calories per 4 tablespoons.

▶ **Formulas** Most infants are given formulas made of either evaporated or whole milk. There are many other excellent prepared formulas on the market to which only water need be added. (See FORMULAS.)

▶ **Supplementary Foods** Vitamins are generally added to the infant's diet at about three weeks of age. There are many standardized excellent multiple vitamin preparations available. They contain 50 mgm. of vitamin C, so that it is not absolutely necessary to introduce fruit juice (orange juice) at this time.

▶ **Solid Foods** Many infants are very hungry at birth, and frequently it may be necessary to introduce cereal, vegetables, fruits as early as 6 weeks to 2 months. However, *not all infants will tolerate the addition of these new foods.*

▶ **Frequency, Quantity, Burping** The frequency and amounts of feeding at each meal vary in all infants. There is now general agreement that a modified self-demand schedule satisfies most children better than a rigid time-clock schedule. This is also easier on the mother. Small infants of six pounds tend to eat every two or three hours because their capacity is small. As they gain weight, they will tend to get hungry at longer intervals. Up to two months of age, six or seven feedings may be necessary.

After the second or third month, the 2 A.M. feeding is usually discontinued with most babies. The total fluid intake does not have to exceed more than thirty-two ounces per day, and the maximum fluid per meal does not have to be greater than eight ounces. If the entire amount is not taken in the form of milk, it can be provided with water (sweetened or unsweetened), juices, and fluids diluted into the cereals and solid foods.

Burping or bubbling the infant is necessary to get rid of gas or air which accumulates in the stomach. If this is not done, the air may cause discomfort, cramps, and mechanical vomiting. The latter is readily seen when the child brings up a great deal of food along with a large amount of gas. In these cases, it may be necessary to burp the baby before and, frequently, during a feeding, as well as afterwards.

When the infant weighs approximately twelve to fifteen pounds, regular whole milk may be substituted for formula feeding. In areas where water is purified and sanitation modern, sterilization of bottles and boiling of water may be discontinued when the baby is six weeks to two months old. In periods when the child has diarrhea or is ill with some gastrointestinal disturbance it may be necessary to go back to sterilizing bottles.

▶ **New Foods** New foods should be introduced gradually, preferably one at a time for a few days, to see whether there is any adverse reaction. It may be necessary to mix the vegetables and meats with a little water to make them more fluid so that the child can swallow them more easily. A toothless infant cannot manipulate sticky or pasty foods. He is accustomed to swallowing liquids and may reject undiluted solids. Following is a schedule of approximate ages for the introduction of new solid foods:

6 weeks to 3 months. Introduce precooked cereals, mashed banana (fresh or canned), some vegetables or other fruits.

4 months. Introduce cooked cereals, fruits, vegetables, hard-boiled egg yolk.

5 months. Introduce meat soups (chicken, bouillon, beef broth), pureed vegetables, meats.

6 to 8 months. Introduce whole milk, zwieback, puddings, custards, cheese.

8 to 12 months. The child may go on 3 meals a day—hard-boiled egg white may be introduced first, then boiled egg with the white incompletely cooked may be tried.

12 to 18 months. The child may eat most adult foods except fish with bones.

"Junior" foods, or chopped foods, are often refused until the child has sufficient teeth to chew lumpy masses. Since such food is just as nutritious in strained form, there is no particular advantage in forcing junior foods before the child is willing to accept them. Fillet or canned salmon and tuna fish may be used as protein substances.

Some children are allergic to cow's milk protein. This may show up as a series of digestive disturbances characterized by diarrhea, vomiting, intestinal cramps and colic, rash, a general irritability and disagreeableness. There are many non-allergenic milks made from soybeans. Your doctor will advise you whether it is necessary for your child to switch to this type of milk. Another form of milk, good for digestive disturbances, is lactic acid milk. Powdered protein milks are often used for the treatment of intestinal disturbances and for the feeding of premature infants.

INFLUENZA   Influenza, or "flu," is a virus disease which occurs in epidemics, generally in the winter and spring. The usual symptoms are the sudden onset of muscular aches, headache, fever, and symptoms referable to the respiratory tract, such as nasal stuffiness, sore throat, and dry cough. The illness generally lasts for some days. The flu is noted for producing a prolonged period of debility, many victims feeling weak and sub-par for some weeks. The fever during the first few days may be on the order of 101°-102°F., and occasionally even higher. It generally abates within three days but occasionally may last longer.

Treatment. None of the known antibiotics are of value in treatment. Probably the most useful drug is aspirin, one to two tablets four times a day, which lowers the temperature and relieves much of the aching. For severe headache small doses of codeine or a similar pain killer may also be used. An alcohol sponge bath may be of value for high fever. Epidemics in recent years have indicated that elderly individuals, patients with chronic heart or lung disease, and pregnant women are more susceptible to flu, and a higher death rate has been reported in these three groups. Immunization against flu, using a vaccine made of several strains, should be given to susceptible individuals and pregnant women. The immunization lasts for only a year and must be repeated at the start of each respiratory season.

There are a large number of viruses which can produce other respiratory illnesses which are also sometimes called flu or grippe. These produce less muscular aching, less fever (as a rule), and more head-cold symptoms. True influenza has no particular effect on the digestive tract. It only rarely causes nausea or vomiting, and does not produce diarrhea.

INSOMNIA   Inability to fall asleep, light slumber with repeated episodes of wakefulness, or early morning awakening with inability to go back to sleep comprise some of the forms of insomnia. Sleep difficulties are not uncommon, especially toward the end of pregnancy; abdominal enlargement may interfere with restful positioning and turning, and there seem to be times in the quiet of the night when the thrashing about of the unborn baby seems to be almost deliberately intended to keep the mother awake. Hot weather may further add to the difficulties encountered.

Sometimes psychological factors such as worry, anxiety, or fear may lead to insomnia. Having a baby often changes a woman's sleep patterns temporarily if not permanently. New babies are notoriously unaware of day-and-night differences. The need for 2 A.M. feedings may not be bypassed for some months, while older babies may regularly wake at 5 A.M., fresh and playful. These interruptions of sleep do not constitute insomnia, although some mothers complain of difficulty in going back to sleep once they have been up.

There is often no wholly satisfactory answer to the insomnia problem. Among the suggested solutions are: (1) A warm (not necessarily hot) tub bath. (2) A light meal or a glass of warm milk shortly before retiring; occasionally beer or wine may produce sleepiness. (3) A whole host of drugs, which are not barbiturates (the classical sleeping pills) may prove of use. Even mild ones may be adequate. They include antihistamines—the drugs used for allergic reactions—which are mildly sleep-inducing, the oldtimer phenobarbital, meprobamate (Miltown®, Equanil®), Doriden® and many others. (4) The standard sleeping pills include Seconal® (red), Nembutal® (yellow), sodium amytal (blue), Tuinal® (blue and red), Carbrital® (white with a blue band), and various others; they can be secured only on a doctor's prescription. For temporary use there is certainly no major objection to any one of these. Their use should, however, be discouraged in favor of other possibilities. Nevertheless, as many weary victims of insomnia, and their doctors too, will point out, one thing worse than taking a sleeping pill is insomnia. Tranquilizers or psychotherapy may be better solutions than barbiturates.

INTELLIGENCE AND MENTAL RETARDATION

▶ **Intelligence Tests** *The Wechsler Intelligence Scale* is made up of ten tests, each testing a different process of intellectual functioning. Five of these sub-tests are *verbal*, which means that the child answers questions on the tasks presented to him. The other five are *performance* tests, which means the child manipulates materials in order to solve the tasks presented to him.

The verbal sub-tests test information, comprehension, arithmetic, similarities, vocabulary, and digit span. Similarities test the formation of concepts. This relates to the ways in which similar things belong together, such as a pear and an apple, which are both fruit. This tests the ability to think in abstractions and is often interfered with by organic brain damage. In another test, the child repeats series of digits which become progressively longer. This gives a measure of his ability to maintain continuous concentration and retain units of information and their relationships.

On the performance sub-tests, the picture arrangements sub-test is a series of pictures which the child is asked to rearrange so that they make a meaningful story. This test measures planning, anticipation, and the ability to see relationships between events.

The picture completion sub-test consists of twenty drawings which are presented one at a time, and the child is asked to tell what important element is missing in each drawing. This tests the child's ability to discover inconsistencies and incompleteness.

The block design sub-test consists of seven geometric designs; the child is asked to assemble colored blocks of wood so that they reproduce a specific design. This test measures visual-motor coordination. It utilizes two intellectual processes; the child must first differentiate the pattern into its parts, then must take these parts and reassemble the design. This particular sub-test is designed especially to test brain-damaged children. Those who have organic brain damage show great difficulty with this test.

The object assembly sub-test consists of four puzzles which the child is asked to assemble. This is also a measure of visual-motor coordination. Children who fail in this test are unable to determine the correct interrelationship of the parts.

The coding sub-test tests the ability to maintain correct spatial relationships while transporting a mental symbol. Brain-damaged children frequently reverse or invert symbols when copying them. It is another test of visual-motor coordination.

The Bender Motor Gestalt Test is a series of eight geometric designs presented to a child who is asked to copy them on a sheet of paper. This tests the ability to perceive order and organize the parts of a design and their interrelationship, and to reproduce this design. It is basically a visual-motor coordination test, but also tests other psychological functions. Brain damage is frequently diagnosed by failures in this test.

The Rorschach Test is a series of ten ink blots printed on ten cards—five in black-and-white and five in color. The child is asked to look at each of these designs and tell what it looks like, or what it reminds him of. This test shows up conflict areas, impulses, personality devices, and the ability of the child to integrate and make use of information. It is helpful in diagnosing neurologically damaged children.

The Thematic Apperception Test. Here the child is shown pictures of either humans or animals in various situations and is asked to tell a story about what is going on in the picture. These tests provide information on how the child sees himself, his environment, and his relationship with others.

▶ **Mental Retardation (Feeblemindedness)** The intelligence quotient (I.Q.) is a convenient and descriptive numerical device for defining intelligence. The intelligence quotient is arrived at by dividing the child's mental age (derived after tests) by his chronological age and multiplying the result by 100.

An average or normal I.Q. is between 90 and 110. A score above 130 indicates superior intelligence, and one above 140, very superior intelligence. Idiots have an I.Q. range from 0 to 20, and they do not develop beyond a mental age of 3. Imbeciles' I.Q. is 20 to 50. These never develop beyond a mental age of 3 to 7. Morons' I.Q. is 50 to 70. These do not reach a level higher than age 10 or 11.

Causes of mental retardation. Mental retardation is only a symptom of poor development of various mental faculties, and may be caused by many different conditions. Heredity, neurological diseases, virus or other infections in the mother (German measles, toxoplasmosis, syphilis), Rh incompatibility, endocrine disorders (cretinism), and chromosome abnormality (mongolism) are some causes of mental retardation.

Birth trauma, hemorrhage in the brain, lack of oxygen immediately following birth, etc., may also cause developmental abnormalities resulting in defective intelligence.

After birth, infections of the nervous system, such as encephalitis, convulsions, meningitis, brain trauma (fractured skulls), etc., may also cause retardation. Severe emotional disturbances, and lack of proper training and of mental stimulation may retard mental growth temporarily.

JAUNDICE Jaundice is a yellow discoloration of the skin and eyes produced when red blood cells disintegrate; they release hemoglobin which is changed to bilirubin (a bile pigment). This causes the yellow color.

Physiologic jaundice (icterus neonatorum) occurs during the first few days of life. There is increased destruction of red blood cells and decreased excretion of the bile pigment by the infant's immature liver. The jaundice usually appears from the second to the fourth day and disappears by the seventh or fourteenth day. This jaundice is perfectly normal and is seen in about 40 per cent of all newborn infants. There is no associated enlargement of the liver or spleen. The blood tests are normal in this condition.

However, there are a few other conditions at birth which cause jaundice due to abnormalities.

1. *Malformations of the bile tract,* such as stenosis of the common bile duct, or absence of the hepatic or common ducts, may cause obstruction and jaundice. A plug of bile or mucus in the common bile duct may also cause obstruction. In this condition, the jaundice may occur at birth or a few weeks later. The liver is usually enlarged and stools may be clay colored. Special blood tests and X-rays are necessary to confirm it.

2. *Syphilitic jaundice.*

3. *Sepsis with jaundice.* This is a condition of severe infections with organisms causing marked toxicity and jaundice.

4. *Erythroblastosis fetalis* (Rh disease). This is a hemolytic disease of the newborn. It is due to the fetus (baby in uterus) producing antibodies to the RH negative blood cells of the mother.

5. *Icterus praecox.* This is a mild form of hemolytic disease of the newborn due to ABO blood-group incompatibility between the mother and infant. It resembles erythroblastosis. Transfusion with Group O blood is usually necessary. It occurs in first-born infants, whereas erythroblastosis fetalis occurs mainly in subsequent births.

Other causes of jaundice are infectious mononucleosis, Cooley's anemia, infectious hepatitis, sickle cell anemia, and acute hemolytic anemias, either congenital or acquired.

LARYNGITIS   Inflammation of the larynx (voice box) is commonly seen in various respiratory infections. The most common symptoms are huskiness of voice, weakness of the voice—it can be reduced almost to a whisper—cough, and, frequently, sore throat. Other parts of the respiratory system may be affected so that there may also be stuffy nose, sinusitis, or perhaps bronchitis with cough and phlegm production.

There is no prompt cure for laryngitis; most of the trouble is due to inflammatory swelling, which even under the best of circumstances may take several days to disappear.

Treatment. Various measures that are helpful are: (1) Voice rest. In severe cases there may be an absolute ban on speaking and the victim may have to communicate by using pencil and paper. (2) Antibiotics may or may not be used, depending on whether the symptoms are considered to be primarily viral or not. Purely viral inflammations do not as a rule respond to antibiotics. (3) Maintaining high humidity in the room by having a vaporizer going or placing pans of water on radiators is soothing. By contrast, inhalation of very dry hot air may be irritating. (4) Hot drinks, often tea or tea-and-honey mixtures, may allay soreness and coughing. (5) Cough may be an annoying symptom and in itself may tend to keep the larynx irritated. Cough suppressants such as codeine or related medicines may then be of value.

Chronic laryngitis is very often due to excessive cigarette smoking. The symptoms may be much like those described above, except they are not associated with respiratory infections and tend to persist the year 'round. Finally, polyps and other growths on the vocal cords, most commonly seen in the middle-aged, may produce hoarseness and voice weakness and thus simulate laryngitis.

LEGS, SWELLING OF Swelling of the legs is generally due to accumulation of fluids in the skin which results in a puffiness, easily demonstrated by pressing firmly with a finger. This will leave a dent which will fill in only slowly. When marked, it is called dropsy, but is generally referred to by physicians as edema.

A variety of causes, mostly not at all serious, may produce swelling of the legs. In pregnancy it is due to pressure on the great veins bringing the blood back from the lower extremities. When present, varicose veins may also contribute, since they are not effective in bringing blood back to the heart. In addition, in pregnancy the great amounts of hormones that are secreted tend to increase the edema. Considerable amounts of salt will always aggravate any tendency to such swelling.

Apart from the various circulatory disorders of the veins mentioned above, the circulatory changes produced by weak-

224

ness of the heart muscle may produce edema. Marked swelling may result. The condition generally requires treatment with digitalis, which strengthens the heart, and with diuretic drugs which promote the excretion of fluid from the system.

Various disorders of the kidneys may underlie some cases of leg swelling. Any disorder which leads to a significant loss of albumin into the urine will lower the amount of this substance present in the blood. One of the sequels to this is that some of the fluid normally kept within the bloodstream will tend to diffuse out into the tissue so that puffiness results. Such edema due to kidney disease may produce obvious puffiness of the hands and of the face, in contrast to that found in heart disease which tends to be limited to the lower extremities. In the childhood disease known as nephrosis there is general swelling in all the tissues, associated with a marked drop in the albumin of the blood.

Treatment. For swelling due to kidney disease, restriction of salt, diuretic drugs, and other measures are useful. When the swelling is due to local circulatory causes such as those in the veins of the extremities, elastic hose are often useful. Some of these are sold commercially, but they can also be made up to order. By exerting compression on the veins, fluid accumulation is diminished. Keeping the legs elevated as far as possible is a further useful measure.

LONGEVITY   There are important hereditary aspects to longevity. We all know families in which everyone lives to a ripe old age, and the contrary is also known to be true; in trying to evaluate this factor in one's own family, death from such events as accidents, influenza or other infections, operations, or similar incidents or accidents are to be excluded.

Progress in medical science has shed some light on the factors involved in long life, and whether or not longevity runs in one's family, certain important factors have been evaluated. Some of the leading ones follow:

1. *One's sex.* Everything else being equal, women have, on the average, a seven-year-longer life span than men. Mainly this can be ascribed to the fact that a woman's cardiovascular system stands up better because of the protection afforded throughout the first fifty years or so by her own female hormones.

2. *Cigarette smoking.* As with other forms of exposure to toxic substances, cigarette smoking ages the organism. As long ago as 1938 it was shown that heavy smokers lived on the average four years less than non-smokers.

3. *Overweight.* The majority of individuals who reach a ripe old age are slender, sometimes even underweight. A body weight 10 per cent above the desirable range has a significant effect in shortening life, and this effect increases with the degree of overweight. There is an increased incidence of heart attacks, high blood pressure, and diabetes in overweights as compared to normals.

4. *Elevated blood pressure.* More than half of all deaths in the United States are due to disease of the heart and blood vessels; any factor that increases or decreases this will affect many millions of individuals. High blood pressure tends to age the blood vessels and can seriously increase the work of the heart. Hence heart attacks and strokes occur more frequently in hypertensives as compared to normotensives. Combinations of overweight and elevated blood pressure are considerably more serious than either of these conditions alone.

MASTURBATION   Masturbation is a practice of handling one's own genitals for the purpose of sexual excitation and pleasure. It occurs to some degree in all children as part of the general desire to see, touch, and be curious. Since sexual feelings are a normal part of growing up, it is to be expected that sexual exploration and experimentation will occur. Children are not aware that the adult world considers this a shameful or disgusting practice.

Parents should be informed that masturbation is not harmful, will not (as was once believed) cause insanity, and does not in itself have any bad effects. However, if a child is made to feel that such pleasurable activity is completely wrong, sinful, harmful, and that he may be threatened with removal of his organ because of it, it may create a permanent and terrible inhibition regarding sex which will cause a neurosis, or sexual disturbance, in later life.

MEASLES (RUBEOLA)   Contagious.
  Cause. Virus.
  Incubation period. 10 to 12 days.

226

Symptoms. Before the typical spots of measles break out there is a severe cold, frequently with high fever, harsh brassy cough, red eyes and an expression of general misery. The cold does not get better with the usual antibiotics and cough medicines—rather, it seems to get worse until the rash appears. The skin rash is preceded by a rash inside the mouth, called "Koplik's spots." These are tiny white specks, like salt sprinkled on the mucous lining of the mouth, very small and difficult to see without magnification. The rash of measles appears first around the ears and neck, then spreads to the face, arms, and body. They are typical flat, round, red spots, approximately the size of a small split pea. The rash disappears between the fourth and fifth day, fading first where it first appeared. The cough and fever diminish slowly after the rash has reached its full bloom, then the patient improves. Cough may persist, however, and the skin may show some dark pigmented areas and peel.

Complications. Swollen glands, measles pneumonia, ear infections, and sometimes encephalitis (brain fever) may follow measles. Encephalitis is a rare but dangerous complication of measles characterized by high fever, lethargy, delirium, convulsions, and/or coma. The result of severe measles encephalitis may be permanent brain damage.

Treatment. Most simple cases of measles respond to aspirin, cough medicines, soothing skin applications (to relieve itching), and a fluid or light diet. The lights should be kept dim because children with measles find it difficult to look at bright light. Persistence of fever, or cough, after seven to ten days requires the attention of a physician.

Prevention. There are now two measles vaccines available for producing permanent immunity. One is a killed-virus vaccine, the other a live attenuated-virus vaccine. The latter is administered with gamma globulin in order to modify any side effects. In cases where there is not sufficient time after exposure to immunize the child with permanent vaccine, an injection of gamma globulin provides some temporary immunity lasting about a month. It also will modify a severe case if given early enough.

► **German Measles (Rubella)** Contagious.
Cause. Virus.
Incubation period. 14 to 21 days.

227

Symptoms. A general feeling of illness, mild fever, swelling of the glands in the back of the neck and head, followed by a pink rash which appears first on the face, then spreads over the head, arms, and body. It rarely covers the legs. The rash resembles measles the first day, scarlet fever the second; it fades on the third.

The particular danger of this disease occurs when pregnant women get it within the first three months of pregnancy. During this period there is crucial development of certain parts of the developing fetus. It has been observed that when German measles affects the developing fetus, the children are born with various abnormalities, including blindness and deafness.

Treatment. Injections of gamma globulin may be helpful. In cases where the disease is contracted by a woman during the first three months of pregnancy, it is frequently an indication for legal therapeutic termination (abortion) of the pregnancy.

MENOPAUSE   Menopause is sometimes referred to as the "change of life," or the "climacteric." The menopause marks the halt of usual cyclic activity of the ovaries. Production of egg cells (ovulation) and all the accompanying changes in the uterus which mark the menstrual cycle end with the menopause.

The menopause sometimes comes on quite abruptly, but more often is marked by a gradual onset with scantier periods, and skipping of periods. A frequent accompanying symptom is hot flushes (flashes)—a circulatory disturbance in which a wave of heat is felt, most often over the face but sometimes over a larger part of the body. This is frequently accompanied by a transient sweat and obvious flushing. Hot flushes occur erratically (sometimes many times a day) and may be increased by emotional upset, weather fluctuations, fatigue, etc. Onset of the menopause is variable; it may occur as early as the late thirties, as late as the mid-fifties. A diagnosis of the menopause cannot be made so long as a woman is menstruating regularly. Thus, a woman in her forties who is still menstruating is wrong to ascribe irritability, depression, joint pains, changes in blood pressure, etc., to the menopause.

Treatment. When menopausal symptoms are severe and the menopause occurs very early, the doctor may well advise the

228

taking of female hormones. There is no reason to fear the possibility, once raised, that taking such hormones might increase the number of tumors in the female reproductive tract; indeed, quite to the contrary, some doctors hold that women should continue female hormones at some dosage level since this protects them against aging changes in the blood vessels and bones.

There has been an increasing tendency in recent years to give women female hormones if they go into an early menopause, or if a heart attack has been experienced. The routine very often is to prescribe the hormones for about three weeks at a time, to be alternated with a period off the drug. This may result in the appearance of a menstrual flow similar to, though perhaps scantier than, that which the woman previously experienced.

One of the reasons for permitting menstruation to occur in this way is that by the shedding of the uterine lining an unduly prolonged hormonal stimulation is avoided. The artificial cycle thus imitates natural ones, just as, in women who take the birth-control pills, stopping the pills will generally result in a menstrual flow several days later. Occasionally, in women taking these hormones, a pink staining may appear which resembles a light flow. This is known as "break-through bleeding" and may be an indication for increasing the dose of the drug for at least a short period. There is much current discussion on this matter; it is conceivable that a medical opinion will eventually favor extended use of hormones, which will thus abolish the menopause.

MENSTRUATION AND OVULATION

▶ **Menstruation** The formation of an egg in the ovary is associated with hormone secretions which produce a cycle of growth and development in the lining of the uterus (womb). If the egg is fertilized and pregnancy initiated, the fertilized egg will implant itself in the uterine lining which has been especially prepared to receive it. In the absence of pregnancy much of the prepared lining is cast off to the accompaniment of bleeding, a process termed menstruation.

Many aspects of menstruation are subject to variability. Although the interval is generally supposed to be twenty-eight days, many perfectly normal women have cycles which are definitely shorter or longer—for example, twenty-four day or thirty-five day cycles. Even greater irregularity may be associated with normal fertility. A nervous upset, a trip, worry over a possible pregnancy, a variety of illnesses, all may lead to a postponement of the menstrual period or even a complete skipping of the cycle. Some women regularly menstruate for only two days, others for seven or more, and the amount of the flow may similarly be quite variable. Adolescent girls frequently have menstrual irregularities, but with the passage of years more regular patterns tend to be established. Definitely scanty periods are referred to as oligomenorrhea, frequent periods as polymenorrhea, painful periods as dysmenorrhea.

Dysmenorrhea generally takes the form of painful cramps, particularly on the first day or two of menstruation. In addition, many women complain of such other symptoms as heaviness and congestion in the pelvic area, backache, and a subpar feeling—"being unwell." Menstrual cramps may be helped by a hot-water bottle, antispasmodic drugs such as are used for disorders of the digestive tract, aspirin and other pain killers, including one useful combination which incorporates small doses of benzedrine with aspirin.

▶ **Ovulation** Ovulation is the release of an egg cell from the ovary; it is the basic event of reproduction. Failure to ovulate (which is rare) will, of course, produce sterility. Ovulation most often occurs about mid-menstrual cycle. Where the length of menstrual cycles is variable, there is evidence that the variability is due to fluctuations in the time before ovulation occurs. Thus ovulation may occur as early as the eighth or ninth day in a short cycle, and as late as the eighteenth or nineteenth day in a longer one. The interval between ovulation and menstruation is considered to be less variable, most often about two weeks. Ovulation generally occurs without a woman having any awareness of it. A few women do experience a lower abdominal pain, which has been termed *Mittelschmerz.*

Ovulatory pain can sometimes imitate appendicitis. It is often associated with bloating and an increased amount of vaginal secretion, which may be pink-tinged. When ovulation produces a definite discomfort, it may be useful to take note of this on a menstrual calendar. An exceptional woman may

230

be able to base her family planning on the regular occurrence of mid-cycle pain or other discomfort. Women who take their temperature every morning for sterility studies will note a slight drop in mouth temperature at about the time of ovulation; this is succeeded by a rise which is maintained in a steady fashion until the time of menstruation. The mid-cycle temperature drop, followed by a rise, may also be a useful indicator of the probability of ovulation.

MONONUCLEOSIS, INFECTIOUS   This disease, which is probably caused by a virus, is of low-grade contagiousness. The incubation period is about four to fourteen days and it is rare in infancy.

Symptoms. The symptoms are fever, swollen glands, signs of upper respiratory infection, sometimes a rash. There may be more severe symptoms with headache, blurred vision, mental confusion, etc. The most important laboratory finding is a large number of abnormal lymphocytes in the blood smear. Another test which confirms the diagnosis is that of a high heterophil antibody titer.

Treatment. The condition lasts about two to four weeks and there is no specific treatment except for general supportive measures.

MUMPS (EPIDEMIC PAROTITIS)

Cause. Virus.

Incubation period. 2 to 3 weeks.

Symptoms. There is painful swelling of the salivary glands, mainly the parotids which are located in the cheeks. Frequently the glands under the tongue and under the jawbone may be involved. The swelling may be on one or both sides and begins just in front of the lobe of the ear. Eating becomes painful because saliva, which is produced during chewing, irritates the gland. This may be noted particularly when sour or tart foods (juices and pickles) are eaten. There is usually fever, headache, vomiting, and lack of appetite, although some cases may be very mild and show none of these symptoms.

Complications. There may be swelling of the sex glands during the first week of mumps, but this rarely occurs in children under twelve to fifteen. If it occurs in males, it may produce sterility. In females, both adult and adolescent, the

231

ovaries may become inflamed and this will produce lower-abdominal pain and tenderness without, however, causing sterility.

Occasionally a neurological complication such as encephalitis may occur. This is characterized by headaches, vomiting, irritability, or lethargy. A physician should always be called for this complication.

Treatment. For mild cases there is no specific treatment except bedrest, aspirin, and soothing or warm applications to the swelling. A bland diet will prevent pain on swallowing or chewing. Swelling is usually over within five to seven days.

Prevention. Injection of a mumps hyperimmune serum is available. It will prevent mumps temporarily (for about a month). In children, mumps is usually such a mild disease that routine use of this serum is not common.

Because there are many other conditions which resemble it (glands swollen from tonsillitis, tumors of the parotid gland, etc.), children with mumps should be seen by a physician.

MUSCULAR CONTROL, DISEASES AFFECTING

▶ **Cerebral Palsy** Cerebral palsy is a disorder of the nervous system which produces many complex symptoms. It may be caused by: (1) congenital malformation of the brain (defects occurring in the development of the brain); (2) brain damage from difficult birth (lack of oxygen or brain hemorrhage); or (3) infection of the brain, with damage, after birth (encephalitis or poisoning).

Symptoms. The symptoms vary, depending upon the area of the brain affected and the severity of the damage. The child who doesn't walk, talk, sit, or develop moving abilities may have this condition. It frequently produces spastic limbs. If one limb is involved, this is called monoplegia. In hemiplegia, the arm and the leg on one side are affected. In paraplegia both legs are affected and in quadriplegia all four limbs. Most of the cerebral palsy lesions produce a spasticity (tenseness) of the muscles, so that moving and walking are difficult. About 60 per cent of palsied persons are spastic. In other forms, when the base of the brain is involved, movements may be bizarre, slow and wormlike (athetoid movements). Because of the excess of involuntary movements, these persons may have extreme difficulty in manipulating things with their hands, and in walking.

Treatment. The treatment for this condition is usually rehabilitation and corrective surgery. Sometimes medications are successful in reducing extra movements.

► **Epilepsy** Epilepsy is a disease characterized by recurring attacks of convulsions. Sometimes the disorder is a hereditary one, while other cases may be of acquired origin. Tumors or brain disease (damage) may cause secondary convulsions. "Grand mal" is a major seizure, followed by tonic and clonic spasms of the arms or legs associated with loss of consciousness. There may be a warning (aura) that the attack is about to occur. This may come in the form of sensations of light, sound or smell.

"Petit mal" is a milder form of the same disease, and is characterized by minimal temporary loss of consciousness. The head may drop, and the patient may appear to be staring blankly.

Neurological investigation should be done in all cases of convulsions. The electroencephalogram, which records brain waves, may determine the specific type of epilepsy present. There are many drugs which will prevent epileptic seizures, without actually curing the disease.

► **Muscular Dystrophy, Progressive** This is a hereditary and familial disease characterized by progressive weakness and wasting of the muscles. There is difficulty in learning to stand or walk, then a waddling gait due to weakness of the muscles of the buttocks. Persons with this disease fall frequently and have difficulty coordinating their movements. A typical feature of muscular dystrophy is the inability to rise steadily to a standing position from a sitting one on the floor. Physiotherapy and general supportive measures are important, but there is no specific treatment for this condition.

NAUSEA AND VOMITING   A great many disorders may produce symptoms of nausea and vomiting. During pregnancy symptoms of this kind characteristically occur in the morning but are very variable, and some women seem to escape them altogether. (See CHILDBIRTH AND PREGNANCY, Morning Sickness.) Other common causes are food poisoning, certain viral or infectious diseases, overindulgence in alcohol, some disorders of the inner ear, and a whole range of disorders involving the upper digestive tract. Among the latter are ulcer, tumors, functional spasms, and reaction to some drugs such as aspirin in overdosage as well as to the heart medicine digitalis. Migraine often produces nausea and vomiting, hence the term "sick headache." Obviously many of these conditions will require a doctor's diagnosis and advice. When the cause is an obviously temporary one, the chief practical problem will revolve about the procedures that will make the transition back to normal easiest.

Treatment. There are some drugs which will diminish or do away with nausea, and some of these (as in the case of seasickness remedies) are available over-the-counter. Small doses of sedatives or tranquilizers will usually help diminish nausea. Other points to be kept in mind are the following: (1) Only small amounts of liquid should be taken at a time. Sudden distention of the stomach, even drinking only a cupful of tea, may provoke another bout of vomiting. Small frequent sips will be better. (2) Sucking on chips of ice may help, and sips of a cold carbonated beverage, such as ginger ale or a cola drink, may be retained when other items are not. (3) Small doses of cola syrup at ten-to-fifteen-minute intervals may often stay down and seem to have a sedative effect on the stomach. Check this treatment and the dosage with your doctor.

Once it is clear that small quantities of such fluids are being retained, one can cautiously expand to somewhat larger quantities and start adding solids. Small amounts of bland cereals such as farina or oatmeal are very commonly employed after gastrointestinal upsets. These can be followed by toast with jams or jellies, small amounts of eggs or milk (only if the patient likes them, however); as performance improves, chicken, potatoes, various soups, chopped meats and the like can be added.

▶ **Vomiting in Infancy** Vomiting occurs in many illnesses. It may be one of the first symptoms of any febrile disease (a disease accompanied by fever). A child may appear perfectly well and then suddenly vomit a meal. This is an indication that the temperature should be checked, as he may be developing some illness. Excess air-swallowing, too rich a formula, indigestion from foods introduced too early, may all cause vomiting. Conditions of the intestine such as abdominal obstruction (blocking of the passage of food) may cause vomiting.

Emotional and psychological factors in vomiting are common causes. If a child is very angry or disturbed, is punished or scolded during a meal or shortly afterwards, this may cause him to become so upset he will vomit his food.

A child may have no fever at the onset of vomiting. However, if the temperature is checked within an hour or two and is rising, this may give some indication of oncoming illness.

Congenital defects in the abdomen, such as pyloric stenosis, cause a persistent projectile vomiting within the first seven weeks of life. This condition can usually only be relieved by surgical operation.

NECK, STIFFNESS OF   What is generally referred to as "stiff neck" is a musculoskeletal condition, generally temporary, which produces pain and tightening-up of a neck muscle. Sometimes the painful spasm of the neck muscle makes it stand out quite prominently and even throws the neck to one side, a condition known as "wry neck," called torticollis by medical men. Any of a considerable number of stresses, torn fibers, or inflammations involving the bones, ligaments, or muscles of the neck may underlie this complaint.

A stiff neck is sometimes noted in the morning on awakening, and a person may be aware that he has slept with his neck at an uncomfortable angle, perhaps off the pillow. Drafts or exposure to cold and dampness may also produce a stiff aching muscle in the neck region. A stiff painful neck may come on almost instantly after certain kinds of twisting motions, as in athletic contests; this is comparable to the acute lumbosacral strains (low backaches) which can arise from as simple a motion as leaning over to pick up a shoe. Probably the twisting motion of the spinal vertebrae produces a slippage between their facets or a slight tear in some of the ligamentous fibers running between them. A painful spasm of the nearby muscles, designed by nature to prevent further motion, will then be the result. Many of these acute painful conditions of the neck last for several days.

Stiffness of the neck is also seen in meningitis and poliomyelitis as well as several other disabling diseases, including infection or irritation in the central nervous system. In these diseases, fever and other evidences of a general infection differentiate the condition from muscular or arthritic involvement of the neck region.

Treatment. The usual treatment for a musculoskeletal condition may include manipulation or stretching, ointments or liniments that produce local heat (known as counterirritants), hot compresses or a heating pad, aspirin, or other pain-killing drugs. (See also POLIOMYELITIS.)

NEUROLOGICAL CONDITIONS

Some of the commoner forms of neuritis follow:

1. *Shingles* is produced by the herpes zoster virus, which is related to the viruses of chicken pox and cold sores. It generally affects a single nerve on one side, most often on the trunk. It produces a patchy or bandlike eruption usually with severe burning pain and exquisite tenderness.

2. *Bell's palsy* affects the facial nerve and produces a characteristic weakness and drooping of the lower side of the face around the lips. Since no sensation is transmitted by this nerve, only the muscle weakness will be complained of.

3. *Sciatica* affects the largest nerve of the body, the sciatic. There is usually pain along the course of the nerve, and a mixture of disordered sensations and muscle weakness. The common causes include the pressure of disks or of the bony spurs produced by arthritis, and inflammations.

4. In *polyneuritis,* many nerves are involved due to a generally acting rather than a local cause. The long nerves going to the limbs are usually the more seriously affected. Pain and weakness are the common complaints. The muscular weakness can lead to inability to raise the wrists or the feet—wrist-drop and foot-drop.

Treatment. To treat neuritis properly one must ascertain the cause. Shingles and Bell's palsy may be helped by steroids. Sciatica may be helped by bedrest, and sometimes traction on the lower spine is employed. Neuritis of nutritional origin is treated by large doses of the vitamins. A traumatic neuritis such as may occur with a fall or a fracture may simply require the passage of time for recovery, but in general neuritis tends to heal slowly.

MULTIPLE SCLEROSIS (MS) MS is a chronic, progressive disease of the central nervous system causing neurological symptoms; such as, difficulty in walking (major cause of disability), speech disorders, mental changes, sensory loss, and visual disturbances. In some individuals, symptoms progress to tremors and complete paralysis. It is estimated that one-quarter of a million Americans have MS with approximately 200 new cases diagnosed every week. Onset manifests itself in early adult life and is frequently associated with sexual dysfunction and urinary problems.

MS is the third most common cause of severe disability between ages 15 and 50 years. The cause is unknown, and there is no cure of specific treatment that will arrest the disease. Medications such as ACTH and corticosteroids may shorten the length of an acute exacerbation, but these drugs do not appear to alter the long-term course. There are no agents that will restore damaged nerve tissues or fibers and their functioning. Multiple Sclerosis appears to be an autoimmune disease in which the immune system is misdirected and turns against healthy body tissue, namely, the myelin sheath that surrounds nerve axons. To date, the best available treatment for MS patients is in symptomatic intervention (treatment to alleviate symptoms as they occur).

The long course of MS may span 30 years or more from onset to death.

NOSE, CONGESTION OF THE

Nasal congestion is common with the common cold; hence many individuals often misdiagnose their nasal congestion as being evidence of a "head cold." There are many other causes including:

1. *Hay fever.* In this condition a hypersensitivity reaction to pollens may produce intense nasal congestion, clear watery discharge, tearing and itching of the eyes. Depending upon the pollens to which the person is allergic it may be experienced in the spring (trees and grasses), in the late summer (ragweed), etc.

2. *Allergies* to dusts, molds, danders (especially of cats and dogs) may produce similar symptoms.

3. *Hormone reaction.* A small group of women experience nasal congestion, sometimes quite intense, during pregnancy. It is considered to be a reaction to hormones whose amounts are increased in pregnancy.

4. *Vasomotor rhinitis.* This is regarded as a functional disturbance which is often made worse by psychologic stress. In some tense individuals the condition is often chronic. The symptoms in many ways resemble those of nasal allergy but can occur at any time of year. It may be seen in children as well as in adults, but often does not come on until middle age.

5. *Physical allergy,* or reactions to changes in temperature or humidity, may set off nasal congestion. Thus some individuals show marked nasal reactions to humidity and to chilling.

Treatment. Despite the varied origins of these kinds of nasal swelling, many persons will show at least some useful response to antihistamines. Thus the running nose and stuffiness produced either by a common cold or by hay fever can be improved with the same medication. Some antihistamines may work better than others with a particular patient, and it may well be worth trying several to determine which is most beneficial. Some are put up in long-acting form so that the duration of effect from a single dose may be twelve hours or longer. Many antihistamines produce sleepiness, and individuals who have to drive a car, take an examination, or otherwise remain alert should be cautioned against this. Nose drops can be used sparingly to decrease nasal congestion, whatever the cause; but their overuse may tend to prolong or intensify nasal congestion. Steroid drugs are sometimes given to break up episodes of intense congestion, and sometimes may work in relatively small dosage. Another group of drugs useful in nasal congestion are called the sympathomimetic amines, drugs of the ephedrine-neosynephrine group. They may be combined with antihistamines and taken by mouth. Patients with elevated blood pressure are generally advised not to take such drugs, however. (See also ALLERGY.)

ORTHOPEDIC CONDITIONS

▶ **Club Foot or Talipes Equinovarus** This is a congenital deformity and requires skilled orthopedic treatment. About 90 per cent of uncomplicated club feet can be treated successfully by manipulation and casting. Severe cases may require surgery.

▶ **Flat Feet** This describes a varying degree of flattening of the longitudinal arch of the foot. The arch itself does not develop in children under the age of two and a half. However, since the bones in the child under two are cartilaginous, the foot must be supported in the correct position until he is four or five years old so that the stress on the bones can be changed and any incipient deformity will not progress. The usual treatment for this deformity is a medial heel wedge, either one eighth or one quarter of an inch high. If the child is very heavy, further measures may be required, such as a heel extension along the medial border of the heel.

▶ **Hip, Congenital Dislocation of** This is a disorder occurring more commonly in females than in males, and one which is not usually noticed until the child begins to walk. There is inability to stand and walk properly, and a waddle is prominent. When examining an infant with this condition, abduction, or pulling of the thigh to the side, is painful and difficult. X-rays of the hips are required in order to make an accurate diagnosis. The treatment is placing the hip in a particular position for a certain period until the hip joint becomes normal. If this condition is not noticed until after two years of age, surgery for this deformity may be required.

▶ **Internal or External Rotation of One or Both Feet** This usually involves rotation of the entire lower leg. Children with the condition show toeing in or toeing out. If there is no deformity around the hips, shoes with a proper heel or sole wedge may be used as correctives. If this is not effective, a Denis Browne bar or similar device is utilized. Here the shoes are fastened to a board, with the heels against the lower edge and the feet toed outward or inward, depending upon whether the child is pigeon-toed or slew-footed. These shoes fastened to the splint are to be worn every night for approximately four months. It takes about five or six weeks for changes to appear.

▶ **Knock-knee** Knock-knee is a condition in which the knees touch and the legs flare, giving the appearance of bow-legs. This may be due to heredity or to rickets. In the latter case the bones are soft and flexible. Heavy infants often appear to have this condition. Certain congenital abnormalities (achondroplasia) may be one cause. Mild degrees of knock-knee and bow-legs usually correct themselves within the limits of their heredity. Extreme deformities may require braces or surgical correction.

▶ **Metatarsus Varus** This is the condition which consists of a turning-in of the outer border of the foot. It is sometimes called a third of a club foot. The condition may tend to correct itself. However, in moderately severe cases, the application of firm "holding" casts for several three-week periods is the treatment of choice. If the foot straightens out and becomes corrected, the child can wear straight-last, normal shoes.

PALPITATIONS This term is generally applied to sensations of forceful beating of the heart or to such irregularities as skipped beats. Very often both of these sensations are experienced together. Skipped beats are generally described as consisting of a beat which occurs somewhat ahead of time in the normal sequence and is then followed by a pause of longer duration than usual. Doctors describe this phenomenon as a premature beat with a compensatory pause. To determine the exact nature of this will generally require an electrocardiogram. In the overwhelming majority of instances, the symptoms described as palpitations are not signs of organic heart disease.

Palpitations occur in some individuals when they have drunk too much coffee or tea, have smoked too much, are excited, under stress or fatigued, or have had insufficient sleep. There sometimes seems to be no identifiable cause: the palpitations may come on abruptly on a particular day, leave as abruptly, and not recur for very long periods.

Far less common than these causes for palpitations, but sometimes described as palpitations, are runs of very fast heart action. The technical name for this is *paroxysmal tachycardia* or *paroxysmal fibrillation*. Such a symptom will certainly need a doctor's attention, and may call for special medication such as digitalis or reserpine. Individuals who can take their own pulse should take careful note of the pulse during these episodes, as such information may be of value to the doctor, especially when the complaint is not present at the time of the office visit.

PLEURISY The lungs and the inner side of the rib cage forming the chest cavity are lined with a thin glistening membrane called the pleura. Inflammation of the pleura is known as pleuritis or pleurisy. Sometimes a fluid is formed which collects around the lung; it is known as a pleural effusion and is sometimes referred to by laymen as "wet pleurisy." With the aid of a little local anesthetic and a needle, the doctor can tap this fluid and examine it, a procedure which may be important for diagnosis. Not all such fluid collections are due to inflammation. A common cause is a weakness of the heart muscle; the resulting congestion may produce a leakage of fluid into the pleural space.

Pleurisy used to be a common accompaniment to old-fashioned lobar pneumonia, where there was often a severe infection of the pleural space known as an empyema. Since the advent of antibiotics empyema has become a rare complication. Somewhat more common are collections of pleural fluid due to virus infections. Some mild inflammations of the pleural lining may result in pain on breathing, though without a significant accumulation of fluid. This is sometimes referred to as pleuritis or "dry pleurisy." Most chest pains that people complain of, including those aggravated by deep breathing, have nothing to do with the pleura or with fluid collections, however. Rather, they arise in ribs or the muscular spaces between the ribs—the intercostal spaces—and pain results when these structures are set in motion on breathing.

Treatment. Pain may be considerably relieved by strapping that part of the chest area with adhesive tape; this produces some immobilization, with resulting relief of pain. Lying on the affected side and taking aspirin or similar pain killers may also be useful. The presence of a collection of fluid in the pleura may indicate different disorders in different age groups, and may well call for a series of diagnostic steps.

PNEUMONIA The bronchial tubes divide and subdivide, finally ending in clusters of air sacs in the lungs. These air sacs are called alveoli, and it is in them that the actual exchange of oxygen between the inspired air and the bloodstream takes place. Inflammation involving the alveoli is called pneumonia or pneumonitis and will produce much more systemic reaction than will bronchitis. The symptoms will generally consist of chills, fever, weakness, shortness of breath, or rapid respiration. Pneumonia may follow bronchitis as the inflammation extends down into the alveoli; this produces a patchy form of inflammation called bronchopneumonia. The classical pneumonia of bygone years, produced by the organism known as the pneumococcus, produced inflammation in an entire lobe of a lung (there are five lobes altogether) and hence was termed lobar pneumonia. Before the introduction of antibiotics, this was a dreaded disease with a high mortality rate.

Rather more common in recent years has been a form of pneumonitis produced by several viruses and referred to as virus pneumonia. Virus pneumonia may involve part or all of the lobe of a lung, usually with some cough, but with relatively little secretion of phlegm. There is usually some fever, but not always, so that sometimes victims of virus pneumonia may be up and about, seemingly not too sick—hence the term "walking pneumonia." In recent years it has been definitely established that the usual organism producing virus pneumonia, the Eaton agent, shows some response to the antibiotic tetracycline. Virus pneumonia can last for some weeks and, like other viral infections, be associated with prolonged debility. In contrast, bronchopneumonias and other pneumonias produced by bacteria usually respond quite promptly to antibiotics, with X-rays showing clearing in a matter of a day or a few days.

POISON IVY   The poison ivy plant produces an acute spreading and weeping eruption of the skin, either by direct or indirect contact with a secretion of the plant. Similar contact irritants are found in poison oak and poison sumac; the skin reactions to all of these are quite similar. Poison ivy tends to spread for a period of some days and produces annoying burning and itching. The involved skin appears red, and little blisters appear which may enlarge and then burst, producing oozing and crusting.

Treatment. Good preventive first-aid treatment following contact with poison ivy is to wash the exposed areas with an alkaline soap, such as yellow laundry soap. If eruption does occur, calamine lotion or lotions containing a chemical called zirconium may be drying and soothing; antihistamines taken by mouth will also help the itching; certain sedative and tranquilizing drugs also have anti-itching properties. For extensive cases of poison ivy, adrenal steroid drugs (cortisone-type drugs) may be taken by mouth or applied locally. They will cut down inflammation and associated symptoms, as well as the tendency of the condition to spread. They are not, however, generally used except for very extensive eruptions in highly sensitive individuals. None of the various attempts to immunize people against poison ivy has proved particularly successful. Individuals known to be sensitive to poison ivy, when exposure to it is unavoidable, should keep all skin areas covered as much as possible.

POISONS AND TREATMENT

POISON	PROCEDURE
ACIDS often fume and are corrosive to tissues.	*Avoid vomiting.* Give large amounts of milk, repeated tablespoon doses of milk of magnesia, or household remedies for heartburn.
ALKALIES produce corrosive burns around lips and mouth. Examples: lye (used in many products for stopped-up drains), ammonia, quicklime.	*Avoid vomiting.* Give large amounts of citrus fruit juices, or diluted vinegar or large amounts of milk.
ARSENIC is found in some ant, mouse and rat poisons, and in some plant sprays. It produces burning stomach pain, thirst, constriction in throat.	*Induce vomiting.* Give large amounts of milk, milk of magnesia, egg whites, or universal antidote.
ASPIRIN is a common ingredient in headache and pain remedies. Poisoning produces flushing, ringing in the ears, gastric irritation, heavy breathing.	*Induce vomiting.* Give bicarbonate of soda (baking soda) in water, one or two teaspoons.
ATROPINE and related drugs (belladonna, hyoscine) are used for spastic disturbances of the digestive tract. Overdosage produces excitement, confusion, dilated pupils, pounding of the heart.	*Induce vomiting,* and alternate with strong tea or universal antidote.

POISON	PROCEDURE
BARBITURATES are found in many sleeping pills and sedatives. Overdosage produces increasing sleepiness, depressed respiration, and coma.	Induce vomiting, unless victim is comatose. Follow with strong coffee. If victim is comatose, give artificial respiration.
CHLORINE is the active agent in various bleaches, produces burning and nausea.	Give milk or emetic and induce vomiting.
CONCENTRATED HOUSEHOLD BLEACHES requiring dilution for use.	Treat as for alkalies.
CLEANING FLUIDS should be checked to see if benzine, kerosene, gasoline, or "petroleum distillate" are present.	Avoid vomiting. Give strong coffee or tea. Artificial respiration may be necessary.
CARBON TETRACHLORIDE or most "spot removers."	Induce vomiting. Give tea or coffee.
CARBON MONOXIDE (motor exhaust fumes) produces headache, weakness, coma.	Give artificial respiration and strong coffee.
DEMEROL (also morphine, codeine, paregoric) is a narcotic, used chiefly as a pain killer. Overdosage produces drowsiness, coma, constricted pupils, and depressed breathing.	Give universal antidote or strong tea. Induce vomiting. If breathing slows markedly, give artificial respiration.
DETERGENTS.	Give milk. Induce vomiting. Repeat with milk and again induce vomiting.

245

POISONS AND TREATMENT

POISON	PROCEDURE
DIGITALIS is a widely-used heart medication. Its derivatives (digoxin, digitoxin, gitaligen) are similar. They produce weakness, headache, slow pulse, collapse, and delirium.	If no more than one half hour or so has passed since taking, *induce vomiting*. Give strong tea repeatedly. Have victim lie down.
FLUORIDES are the active ingredient of many ant and mouse poisons.	*Induce vomiting*. Give large amounts of milk.
IODINE produces stomach and throat pains.	Give any starchy substance—cornstarch, flour, or bread. Then *induce vomiting*.
LEAD, found in some paints and in white and red lead, produces pain in throat and stomach, vomiting, convulsions, collapse.	*Induce vomiting*. Give large amounts of milk or Epsom salts, and *induce vomiting again*.
OIL OF WINTERGREEN is chemically related to aspirin and produces similar symptoms. It is very toxic if swallowed.	Give 1 to 2 teaspoons of baking soda in water. *Induce vomiting*. Repeat the baking soda, and allow it to be absorbed.
PHOSPHORUS, found in roach and rodent poisons, often has a disagreeable garlicky odor.	*Avoid vomiting*. Give half a glass of hydrogen peroxide.
STRYCHNINE is found in rodent poisons.	*Induce vomiting*. Give strong tea and the universal antidote.
TURPENTINE produces burning pain, excitement, weakness, nausea, shock.	*Avoid vomiting*. Give 1 to 2 ounces of Epsom salts in a pint of water.

POLIOMYELITIS (POLIO)   Contagious.

Cause. 3 separate types of viruses.

Incubation period. 5 days to 3 weeks.

Symptoms. Its special symptoms are caused by varying degrees of nerve involvement, with special injury to the anterior horn cells and the motor nuclei of the brain stem. Infections may be caused by one, two, or mixed types, and the symptoms depend almost entirely on the location and severity of the damaged nerve cells. If there is simple injury, the damage may be reversible, and function may return after an initial paralysis.

Polio is classified in the following way:

1. *Abortive.* In abortive cases one sees headache, nausea, sore throat, malaise, and vomiting. These cases are recognized during polio epidemics but do not have muscular or paralytic involvement.

2. *Spinal paralytic.* In this form there is weakness of the neck, trunk, diaphragm, thorax, abdomen, or extremities, due to involvement of the nerves. Preliminary symptoms may occur resembling minor upper respiratory infections, such as headache, sore throat, vomiting, diarrhea, stiff neck, etc. Meningeal irritation and signs of meningitis may occur. There may be muscle pain on extension of the legs and bending of the neck and back.

3. *Bulbar.* In this form, the cranial nerves and centers of breathing and circulation are affected. Symptoms involve the breathing and swallowing mechanisms. Because of moderate paralysis of the swallowing muscles there is difficulty in swallowing fluids, and they may be brought up through the nose. If the breathing center in the brain is involved, paralysis of the muscles of breathing may occur.

4. *Encephalitic.* In this variety there is drowsiness, irritability, disorientation, and tremors. The picture is the same as encephalitis from other causes.

Hospitalization with physical therapy and muscle reeducation are the modern methods of treating polio. In recent years, mass immunization programs with Salk (killed) or Sabin (live attenuated) vaccine have virtually eliminated polio in many countries.

PULSE AND RESPIRATION RATE, HOW TO MEASURE

Pulse rate registers the frequency of the heartbeat per minute. The pulse rate varies in children as well as in adults, and is higher when fever is present. The average normal rate for adults is between 70 and 90 and in children between 80 and 100. In very small infants it can be as high as 110 to 140. The best place for feeling the pulse is directly below the thumb on the wrist. A rapid pulsation will be felt there. If one uses the second hand on a watch, the frequency of the counted beats determines the pulse rate. The rate is recorded as beats per one minute. A pulse rate that is so fast it can hardly be counted is abnormal, and the doctor should be notified. Heartbeat is the same as pulse rate.

Breathing is an automatic function, and we do not regulate or think about it. It just continues. In sick children as in adults, however, the respiratory rate is affected by many factors. Fever, disease, the state of acid base metabolism in the body, all affect the normal rate of respiration which, in adults, is usually sixteen to twenty every minute. In children, it is slightly more frequent. Respiration is counted by observing the number of excursions of the chest per minute. The quality of breathing may also be noted; whether it is regular, irregular, shallow, or deep. It is recorded as breaths taken per minute. The respiratory rate is increased in diseases with fever, such as bronchitis, pneumonia, diabetes, etc. When it returns to normal it is an indication of general improvement. Extremely depressed, infrequent respiration is a serious condition and should be reported to the physician. Respiration rates below ten or twelve per minute are not normal. They may be an indication of impending coma or central nervous system depression. (See also TEMPERATURE.)

RABIES (HYDROPHOBIA)

Cause. Virus.

Incubation period. Varies from 4 to 8 days up to 3 months.

Symptoms. The primary symptom of the nervous system in rabies is that of severe and painful spasm of the muscles of the throat (pharynx and larynx) at the sight of food or liquid. The disease is therefore given the name "hydrophobia," meaning literally, fear of water. Rabies is an acute infectious disease which attacks the nervous system. The virus is transmitted to man by the bite of an infected dog, cat, fox, squirrel, or other wild animal. The virus enters the nervous system and travels by the peripheral nerves to the central nervous system. Degeneration of certain nerves is responsible for the extensive symptoms of spasm, muscle weakness, and finally paralysis. This severe and progressive disease is almost always followed by death. The incubation period of rabies may be much shorter if the bite is around the head and neck. The virus has a shorter distance to travel to the brain.

The symptoms of rabies appear in three phases. The first is characterized by certain peripheral nerve sensations, such as numbness, itching, tingling, and burning, followed by sensations of irritation, restlessness, salivation, perspiration, insomnia, drowsiness, or depression. In the second phase there is excitation. Apprehension and terror appear at this time. The neck may become stiff, and delirium with twitching or convulsive movements may appear. During this second stage, the intensely painful spasm of the throat while attempting to swallow appears. The third phase is represented by increasing paralysis, coma, and death. It is a terminal phase.

Treatment. Rabies in some ways resembles tetanus, but there are many differences. The prognosis for rabies is very poor. Consequently, the best form of treatment is prevention.

Prevention. Most important in preventing rabies is immunizing dogs and other animals who may become contaminated with the virus. If a dog has been bitten by an animal suspected of being infected with rabies, he is either destroyed or isolated for observation to see whether he comes down with the disease. Any animal who has bitten a person should be isolated and observed. Since rabies is such a severe disease, passive immunization with hyperimmune antirabies serum is now an established procedure. Louis Pasteur was the first man to demonstrate the virus in the central nervous system of rabbits, and he developed a vaccine for it.

The immunization treatment against rabies is painful and long. It is therefore important to have all animals and pets immunized against the disease. Bites from animals should be properly cauterized and thoroughly cleansed, and a doctor should be alerted to observe the progress of the case. The antirabies serum should be followed by intramuscular immunization with the vaccine. However, once the disease has developed, all these sera and vaccines are of no value.

RECTUM The last six inches or so of the large intestine is relatively straight and is called the rectum. In a well-functioning digestive tract the rectum may be quite empty except at the time of having a bowel movement. Indeed, the distention of the rectum produced by the movement of stool into it is the usual signal for the need to evacuate, and it is this that the infant has to learn in the course of his bowel training. Inflammation in this area, called proctitis, may also stimulate the desire to move the bowels even though in fact the rectum may be empty.

If the signal to have a bowel movement is neglected, as it may be when people are in a hurry to leave the house in the morning or when it is otherwise inconvenient to have a movement, stool may accumulate in the rectum. Some of its water content may be reabsorbed, thus leading to a hard, dried-out stool such as is seen in constipation. Occasionally (also in weak or bedridden individuals who are unable to recognize or act on the signal for defecation), large amounts of dried-out stool may accumulate in the rectum, which is somewhat distensible. This is spoken of as an impaction. An impaction may necessitate vigorous measures, such as repeated enemas or even removal by hand.

The opening of the rectum is guarded by a circular muscle called the sphincter ani. Paralysis of this muscle occurs in certain conditions and may lead to inability to hold back the stool. One of the rare but distressing tears that may occur in childbirth can also damage the sphincter and lead to difficulty in rectal control. A more common problem, also related to delivery, is a weakening of the muscles of the pelvic outlet which encircle and support the lower rectal region. This may result in the dilatation of the rectum known as a rectocele. Minor degrees of rectocele are of no consequence, but more advanced stages may require plastic surgical repair. Various fluids and medicines may be introduced into the rectum for different purposes—to move the bowels, to soothe local inflammation, or to produce some systemic effect, as when an aminophylline suppository or enema is used in the treatment of asthma.

RHEUMATIC FEVER   Rheumatic fever is caused by the toxic effect of streptococcus infections in children. These tonsillitis and strep throat infections occur more commonly in the spring in the eastern United States and on the West Coast during the winter. The disease may run in families and is also common where there is poverty, malnutrition, and poor hygiene.

Symptoms. The symptoms of rheumatic fever vary, depending on the severity of the infection. The heart and its valves may be involved early, producing characteristic murmurs. In severe cases there is fever, heart murmur, arthritis (inflammation of the joints—generally the ankles, knees, and wrists—with redness and painful swelling). There may be a rash, nosebleeds, abdominal pain, pallor, malaise, and difficulty in breathing. Severe cases may result in heart failure. Laboratory findings in these conditions show a high white blood count and sedimentation rate, typical electrocardiogram, X-ray, and fluoroscopy changes.

Treatment. Rheumatic fever treatment consists of bedrest, antibiotics, sometimes steroids (cortisone). All children who have had rheumatic fever should be placed on preventative treatment with antibiotics to prevent future infections.

Mild attacks of rheumatic fever may go unnoticed and show minimal signs of joint pains and other symptoms. Even with mild attacks, there may be heart involvement. However, the disease may be so mild that it is simply considered inactive rheumatic heart disease. Most patients with acute rheumatic fever should be kept in bed for three to six months. After this they may be permitted out of bed if their blood tests remain normal for two weeks and they look fairly well.

SCARLET FEVER (SCARLATINA)   Contagious.
Cause. Streptococcus.

Incubation period. 2 to 7 days. This is an acute contagious infection, caused by (most frequently) the Group A betahemolytic streptococcus. It may be contracted directly from an active case by droplet infection, or from books, clothing, toys, and other contaminated objects. The incubation period is two to seven days. In the period before the rash breaks out, fever, sore throat, and vomiting usually occur. The temperature may be as high as 104°F. Most cases of scarlet fever occur between the ages of two and eight.

A second attack of scarlet fever usually does not follow the immunity which one attack provides. However, repeated streptococcal infections such as tonsillitis, sinusitis, and ear infections are possible with other strains of streptococcus germs; but a rash does not usually occur with all these diseases.

Symptoms. Children with scarlet fever usually appear very sick. The rash, which resembles red "goose flesh," starts around the neck and chest, spreading over the rest of the body. It is rarely seen on the face. The throat is usually very red, and the tonsils may be inflamed and covered with pus. Glands in the neck are often swollen. At first there is a whitish coating on the tongue; when this disappears, the papillae of the tongue enlarge, leaving what is called a "strawberry tongue." This is a beefy red tongue with tiny swellings (tongue glands). After the height of the eruption (three to seven days) the rash fades and is followed by a slight peeling of the skin.

Complications. Ear, gland, kidney infections, rheumatic fever, and arthritis frequently follow scarlet fever. In recent years the use of penicillin by mouth and by injection has prevented many of these complications. In very severe cases, a convalescent serum can be used.

Immunity. Infants may be immune to this condition up to nine months of age if their mothers are immune. Both convalescent serum and scarlet fever antitoxin may be used to confer immunity. These are not often used; however, permanent immunity may be acquired after having the disease or by five weekly subcutaneous injections of scarlet fever toxin.

Treatment. Children exposed to scarlet fever may be given penicillin or sulfonamides, which may either prevent or at least modify the course of the disease.

SEX EDUCATION   This is a complex subject to cover briefly, and it becomes all the more difficult because of the variability of values and standards of sexual behavior and education in this country. Certain religious groups are very strict about what they consider proper sex education for children. Other psychoanalytically-oriented groups have much more lenient and flexible standards.

The first two or three years of the infant's life are crucial in the development of his feelings. He learns warmth and responsiveness from the way his mother handles him, plays with him, talks to him, feeds and tends him. And he develops an "outgoing" feeling of love and affection, tenderness, and a desire to please and oblige.

Early loving is directed toward the parents, and the children become very attached to them during the first few years of life. Once the child is able to walk and play and have contact with other individuals, he detaches himself a little from his close dependence on the parents and seeks out friendships and affection outside the family circle. Usually sexual feelings go into a "latency" or dormant period until approximately puberty (twelve to fifteen years of age). In the intervening years the child sublimates, or deflects, sexual striving toward other aims, and becomes interested in school, sports, play, and other activities.

The development of sexual feelings is a natural process of growth. Young children make discoveries about their bodies and will frequently experiment with themselves and with each other.

Proper sex information can be given at various stages of the child's life if the parents' attitudes have been "normal." Very often the parents themselves have confused, fearful, guilty attitudes of sin toward sex. These attitudes will often be communicated to the children in the form of shame or punishment. Many parents are too embarrassed to discuss sex matters with their children. A matter-of-fact attitude and a tone of voice which does not unduly indicate disaster in relation to this area of life are the best approaches to take. Children should be informed that sexual and tender, loving feelings should go together. A great deal of sexual difficulty arises when a split exists between sexual feelings and tender, loving feelings. If the parents' ideas and feelings about sex are unclear or uncertain, this will usually be communicated to the children. If discussion regarding this area is too embarrassing or distasteful to the parents, there are books which can be bought for the children, and possibly discussions with the family physician or psychiatrist would be helpful.

SEX ORGANS, FEMALE   The external female sex glands are, together, known as the *vulva*. This includes the larger and smaller vaginal lips, the clitoris, the urinary and vaginal openings, and the hymen. The larger lips (labia majora) mark out the entire vulva. They are essentially folds of skin containing a small amount of fatty tissue, and are covered with hair. Below, they meet and blend into the skin overlying the central area between the vaginal and rectal openings. This central area is sometimes referred to as the perineum. The small lips (labia minora) are two thinner folds of reddish tissue, a good deal smaller than the larger external lips, and are hairless. They meet above in the region of the clitoris, pass downward around the vagina, then blend imperceptibly together below the vaginal openings.

The *clitoris* is a small (perhaps ½ inch), highly sensitive structure with erectile tissue and is analogous to the penis of the male. Stimulation of the clitoris contributes importantly to the pleasure of intercourse. Between the clitoris and the vaginal opening is the urethral opening, the channel for the passage of the urine.

The *hymen* is a rather variable membranous fold at the vaginal opening. In rare cases, a hymen may completely block the vaginal opening, a condition known as imperforate hymen. Usually the hymen will admit at least one finger, occasionally two. It is generally partially ruptured at the time of first intercourse, and only vestiges are left after childbirth.

The *vagina* is an extensible pouchlike structure approximately three to five inches in length, the upper end of which is a blind vault into which the lower portion of the cervix projects. The internal lining of the vagina has a corrugated appearance because of its folds. The walls of the vagina normally lie in contact with one another but are capable of considerable distention, as during intercourse and childbirth. The vagina is kept moist by secretions from the uterus. At its opening are also special glands which secrete a lubricant substance, particularly during sexual stimulation.

In its nonpregnant state the *uterus* (womb) is a small pear-shaped muscular organ. It measures two to three inches in length and consists of an upper larger triangular portion, the corpus, and a lower narrowed cylindrical portion, the neck or cervix. The *cervix* projects into the vagina and there presents a small opening, the *os,* which is the beginning of the canal which runs into the uterus. (In the familiar cancer-detection procedure known as the "Pap" smear, the physician rotates a swab placed just within the os to get a sample of cells.)

Extending outward to the sides of the pelvic cavity and acting as a support for the uterus are membranous folds known as the broad ligaments. Along the upper portion of these ligaments run the *fallopian tubes,* the channels which run from the uterus up to the ovary. Each tube has a trumpet-shaped widening at its ovarian end which receives the egg.

The *ovaries* are almond-shaped structures in which the eggs (ova) are formed. All the eggs of the ovary are present in the newborn female infant, and no more are formed in her lifetime. These tiny structures, known as the primordial follicles, are present by the thousands just below the surface of the ovary; about five hundred of them will come to maturity during a woman's total reproductive lifetime and will discharge a ripe egg capable of being fertilized. At the time of ovulation, one egg bursts out of the ovarian surface and is momentarily free in the abdominal cavity. Apparently, however, it is soon "scooped up" by the fallopian tube.

SEX ORGANS, MALE   The important sex organs of the male are all externally located, in contrast to those of the female. Those internally situated—the *prostate,* the *seminal vesicles*—are of secondary importance. The male external organs are the *penis* (the organ of copulation, whose dimensions vary depending upon sexual stimulation) and the *scrotum* (a container for the *testes*—or testicles—in which the sperm are manufactured). The scrotum is a pouch of skin whose size and appearance is, curiously enough, dependent upon temperature: in hot weather, or after a hot bath, the scrotum hangs quite low and appears smooth and thin-walled; after exposure to cold, it shrinks considerably and has a thicker-walled, corrugated, or wrinkled appearance.

An inadequate erection, or absence of erection in appropriately-stimulating circumstances, will make intercourse impossible and is referred to as impotence. Hostility toward the woman, fatigue, the debility associated with certain illnesses, or neurotic patterns often going back to childhood may contribute to impotence, which may be either a temporary or a long-standing complaint in some men. Aging also plays a part in this diminished capacity to perform sexually, as there is an increasing percentage of impotence occurring in men past forty. Because of the complex psychological features that have a bearing on it, a man may be impotent on one occasion—including even his wedding night—and fully potent on others, when he is less nervous or anxious. A squabble or other marital difficulty may produce the same symptom, although paradoxically it sometimes heightens sexual desire.

The testes are firm, ovoid structures, approximately one and a half inches long. They contain two important groups of cells. One group is in almost constant division, undergoing changes which result in the formation of sperm (spermatogenesis). Not only does this type of change alter a large rounded cell into an elongated whiplike one, but there is at the same time a halving of the total number of chromosomes—from 46 to 23. The second group of cells within the testes secretes a substance called testosterone, referred to as the male hormone. It is this which is related to the increased muscle mass, body hair, and beard of the male, as well as such other features as the heavier bones, the lower-pitched voice, and perhaps some behavioral and psychologic characteristics. Sperm formed in the testicles undergo maturation in the *epididymis* and in the spermatic cord—a pair of channels which runs from the testes through the *inguinal canal* and into the pelvic cavity. Close to the internal portions of the spermatic cords are the *seminal vesicles* and the *prostate,* both of which secrete fluids added to the semen at the time of ejaculation.

► **Undescended Testicles (Cryptorchidism)** Sometimes a boy is born with either one or both testicles undescended. The missing testicle or testicles may have remained higher up in the abdomen, or halfway down in the testicular canal. Frequently, undescended testicles do descend spontaneously into the scrotal sac. If this does not occur by the time the child is six to nine years old, injections of anterior pituitary hormone or testosterone (male sex hormone) are given. Testicles which remain in the abdomen or the canal may become atrophic and result in sterility. If hormone treatment is unsuccessful, surgery is usually necessary.

SEXUAL HARMONY   There is much more to marriage than sex, but a good sexual relationship is a powerful foundation. The sex act can contribute a deep and ever-renewable pleasure; it can allay conflicts, even when nothing is said. Since this is a vital part of marriage, it is unfortunate that even today sex still remains a somewhat taboo topic.

To the extent that sex is not guided by instinct—and in humans instinct is a small part—it is subject to learning and to improvement. Sex education should therefore be looked upon as normal, desirable, and (like a college education) worthy of time and effort. In general, most of the difficulties, and perhaps most of the learning of new lessons, confront the woman. This is not to deny that many men are too hasty and must learn to "slow down," as well as to be more thoughtful or considerate in their approach.

Women often face biological and psychological obstacles to sexual enjoyment. Their sexual drives are more delicately poised and therefore more readily thrown off by fatigue, worry, fear of pregnancy, or other emotions. A fair number of women seem to be unable to achieve an orgasm (climax) even in relatively favorable circumstances. Then, too, there is the lifelong accumulated burden produced by the upbringing which says that sex is not "nice," that a girl should be wary of a man's advances, that a woman cannot be too careful, and so forth. Although there is often a sound basis for these feelings in the young girl emerging into adolescence and in the young unmarried woman, negative feelings about men and sex should not be carried into marriage. The marital state will be happier if more positive feelings toward sexual relationships are developed.

Some common complaints made by husbands are that wives are uninterested, unresponsive, and unwilling. Possibly some men cannot be satisfied with less than a veritable "tiger," while others are simply searching for something that does not exist. Nonetheless, some of the difficulties they complain of *do* exist.

Based on the many things that marriage counselors hear, the following suggestions can be made to the wife: (1) to give freer expression to one's positive feelings—a woman can both speak of and show love in many ways: with a warm (not a routine) kiss, an affectionate caress, the sex act itself; (2) avoidance of a necessarily passive, silent, and acquiescent role in the sexual act—a woman can contribute actively to preliminary love-making as well as to the act itself; (3) demonstration of that "infinite variety" for which Cleopatra was praised—sexual variety can be the spice of life and one should therefore experiment with new approaches and new techniques; (4) recognition that it is not always possible to match up sexual desire—even if a woman's desire is slight on a particular occasion it is still possible to be a loving and responsive partner in the sexual act; and finally (5) when problems *do* come up, one must not hesitate to discuss them with either the husband or the doctor.

▶ **Frigidity** Lack of responsiveness in sexual intercourse, sometimes to the point of absolute distaste, is referred to as frigidity in women. Frigidity is a complex state: it may exist at some times and not at others, and with one man but not another. In many women frigidity may be traced to severe or restrictive upbringing resulting in conscious or unconscious inhibiting feelings of guilt, and poor information or misinformation on the subject of sex. A woman who is brought up to believe that sex is an act of aggression on the part of the man rather than an act of mutual love may find that she is fearful and unresponsive in sexual situations. Also, in our society, there are contradictory attitudes toward sex at all levels. On the one hand, sex is always being emphasized in our entertainment, advertising, movies, and literature. On the other hand, it is simultaneously regarded as "not nice," as an activity that one has to be very secretive about, or as the one major aspect of living that has shameful associations. Were this not so, the fable that it is the stork who brings the baby would not have been invented.

In the more severe degrees of frigidity, fear and hostility always play a part. Fear of the man, fear of being hurt, fear of becoming pregnant may dominate a woman's thoughts and make her sexually unresponsive. If, for one or another reason traceable to her experiences with this or some other man, she has negative feelings toward him, then too she is likely to be frigid. There is little doubt that moderate degrees of frigidity, or at least inhibition about sex, are by no means uncommon among women. However, these inhibitions may be resolved by the progress of a successful marriage and by repetition of successful acts of sexual intercourse. Thus many women who early in marriage fail to experience a climax may do so as they grow more relaxed in the sexual relationship. Often coupled with increased responsiveness on their part is increased expertness on the part of the husband.

At worst, frigidity can break up a marriage; at best, it is bound to be a drag on it. It should, therefore, be dealt with as a serious problem and not be disregarded. The fact that a frigid woman can still have intercourse does not alter the desirability of improving this area of the marital relationship. The problem should be discussed with the family doctor or the gynecologist and, if considered advisable, with a psychotherapist. The great majority of cases of frigidity are susceptible of considerable improvement.

SEXUAL RELATIONS AFTER CHILDBIRTH   As a general rule it can be predicted that there will be no significant changes in the sexual life after childbirth. True, there is first stretching, followed by shrinkage of the various parts. Then there is the healing of the incision which may have been made by the doctor to facilitate childbirth (episiotomy). However, the vagina and adjacent parts will resume their usual dimensions and sensitivity with respect to sexual functioning. A few women may find that the vaginal opening seems tight after an episiotomy. A warm tub and the use of a lubricant will facilitate intercourse for them. As sexual relations are continued the feeling of tightness disappears.

The post-partum discharge, at first red, then white, called the lochia continues for some three weeks. In many women, by the time the lochia clears the usual sexual desires may be experienced. It is generally advised that sexual relations be postponed till the six-week visit to the doctor. In this, as in other matters, one should be guided by one's own doctor's advice regarding resumption of sex. A few doctors believe that sexual relations a bit earlier than this need not fall under an absolute ban, and certainly the husband is not likely to object.

Marked changes in attitude toward sexual relations are generally founded on emotional, not a physical, basis. A woman who has had a difficult pregnancy, a hard labor, and perhaps various kinds of discomfort afterward, may sometimes shrink from intercourse. She may harbor the thought that pregnancy and a new cycle of discomfort may result, even when contraceptive measures are practiced. In a few instances fear of pregnancy and therefore of intercourse may lead to frigidity. It may help such a person if she can be made to understand that with the new birth control pills 100% freedom from pregnancy can be guaranteed. Persistent fear in this kind of situation may require some form of psychotherapy. The reverse may also occur—a woman who has successfully and happily become a mother, is anxious to have more children, and has a good basic relationship with her husband may be more desirous and responsive sexually.

SEXUAL RELATIONS DURING PREGNANCY If all goes well, there is no need for change in a couple's usual pattern of sexual relations during most of a pregnancy. Intercourse may be continued as frequently as formerly, and if the wife is accustomed to having a climax, she may expect to continue to have one. In women with a history of frequent abortions (spontaneous miscarriages), or where there has been bleeding in the presence of pregnancy, sexual relations may be temporarily forbidden by the doctor; in some instances intercourse at about the time when a menstrual period would have appeared may thus be advised against for the first three months. Most doctors also advise that abstinence should be practiced during the last one to two months of the pregnancy. Intercourse is difficult at this time, especially during the last month, and there is a possibility—however remote—of injury or precipitation of labor.

After delivery, it is customary to advise against sexual relations until the six-week checkup visit. Among the contributing reasons for this are the presence of the vaginal discharge (*lochia*) and possibly also a healing *episiotomy*.

Some women experience tightness or pain after the healing of an episiotomy. The liberal use of lubricants may be of help, as is also a preliminary hot tub-bath. If the problem continues, the doctor should be consulted, since gentle dilatation may sometimes be of value. Ordinarily an episiotomy will, if anything, contribute to enhanced sexual gratification.

As a rule, a woman, if nursing her child, will not be likely to ovulate and will therefore remain infertile. The probability is therefore high that she may have intercourse without contraception for at least the first few months of nursing. In the absence of nursing, her fertility will return much sooner; it is quite possible for such a woman to conceive even before she has had her first menstrual period after the delivery. Certainly with resumption of menstruation—i.e., with the first menstrual period—the possibility of a new pregnancy does return.

SHOCK (ELECTRIC)   Most of the electric shocks sustained in the household are not likely to be dangerous unless one is wet and grounded as, for example, when someone standing in the bathtub touches a live electrical outlet. Serious shocks most often result from contact with a main power line which carries high voltages. Contact with such a line may lead to weakness or complete paralysis; unconsciousness may result, together with burns at the contact point.

It is of utmost importance that rescuers should avoid touching not only the line but also the victim so long as the latter is in contact with it. If the line can be switched off promptly, do so! Otherwise push the line away from the victim, using a nonconductive material, such as wood, paper, or rubber. If the victim appears to have stopped breathing, artificial respiration should be started at once; this should be maintained until the doctor arrives, or until the victim is brought to the hospital.

SKIN CARE   The care of the skin is not nearly so complicated as many cosmetic ads intimate. Also contrary to the ads, oiling, creaming, or moisturizing the skin will not prevent such aging changes as wrinkles. Wrinkling is due to changes in the subcutaneous tissue—the connective tissue underlying the epidermis—and agents applied to the surface of the skin will generally have no effect on the underlying connective tissue nor on the unknown and still uncontrolled connective tissue changes that occur with age.

Some women avoid the use of soap and water because they fear a drying effect. The most likely thing that would result from any oversoaping would be a slight flaking of the skin, which in actual fact seldom happens. The skin of the face generally has enough oil glands so that any drying produced by soap is very temporary, and surface film from oily secretion is rather quickly re-formed.

There is no objection to women creaming their faces as a cleansing procedure to substitute for use of soap if it produces no difficulty—it may occasionally lead to a case of acne or seborrhea. The skin of the body, being less oily than the face, *can* be overly dried by soaping. This is seen particularly during the winter, when the amount of secretion is diminished, and the skin tends to be overly dried because of overheated homes. Under these circumstances, in scrupulously clean individuals who like to take an overall soaping daily, some dryness and roughness of the skin with itching may occur. The itching is generally mild and is often referred to as "winter itch." The treatment is to decrease the amount of soaping, to use a soap containing cold cream or a similar agent, or to add oils to the tub or the washcloth. In the older age group particularly, because of decreased oil production, such special measures for replenishing and adding oils to the skin with the bath may be desirable.

▶ **Premature Aging** Probably the most important common factor in prematurely aging skin is excessive exposure to the sun. It has been convincingly shown that all of the characteristic changes that occur in the skin with the aging process are greatly accelerated by overexposure to sunlight. The deep tan developed by the sun worshipper gives a healthy outdoor look at the time, but in the long run will produce an unhealthy, leathery, aged skin. In addition, chronic exposure to the sun greatly increases the possibility of developing cancer of the skin. It would thus certainly be preferable to avoid a way of life of constant sunbathing which increases this likelihood. (The importance of this factor is illustrated by data which show that cancer of the skin of the face is a thousand times more common in Texas than in New York.)

One substance which seems to slow down the aging process in the skin is the female sex hormone. This hormone seems to increase the water content of the skin and decrease aging changes. Various methods of taking advantage of this effect of the female hormone have been tried. One has been to rub female hormone-containing creams into the skin. It has been shown that the hormone will get to the underlying connective tissues and exert an effect there. This approach has been frowned upon because the hormone thus absorbed could have indirect effects on the ovaries of women prior to the menopause, and conceivably on the breasts as well. In recent years, however, there has been a reconsideration of the effects of female hormone, with an increasing tendency to give the hormone to women past the menopause for a variety of sound reasons.

SKIN CARE DURING INFANCY   The newborn child has a skin which is soft, smooth, tender, and velvety. When he is born, he is covered with some blood and a cheesy material called "vernix caseosa." The skin becomes red later; then when it turns lighter again, peeling occurs. It has long been considered axiomatic that every newborn infant required a soap-and-water bath. However, many physicians now realize that the vernix caseosa has a protective character and prevents infections and irritations of the skin if left on for a few days following birth.

When bathing infants, ordinary castile soap may be used. The skin should never be rubbed, but only patted gently. Perfumed soaps are not necessary, and may even be harmful because they may act as irritants and sensitize the skin. It is not usually necessary to use oils on a baby's skin unless it is extremely dry or peeling. Oils produce a blocking of the sweat ducts and glands. They block the bacteria normally found on the skin and produce pustules and clogged glands. Many of the baby oils available contain certain chemicals which either irritate the skin or act as sensitizers.

On the other hand, a mildly astringent liquid, such as pure witch hazel, is cleansing and cooling and does not irritate the skin. Unscented talcum powder may be used instead of fancy perfumed dusting powders. It is now thought best to avoid the use of boric acid as a powder, ointment, or wet dressing. Boric acid is a poison, and instances of death have been reported from its absorption through the skin.

SKIN CONDITIONS AND INFECTIONS

▶ **Acne**   Acne may be regarded as one of the tolls exacted for becoming an adult; unknown in children prior to puberty, acne's onset is associated with sexual development. For reasons not well understood, puberty seems to exert a stimulating effect on the oil glands, chiefly those of the face and upper trunk. The most active hormone in this respect is the male sex hormone; acne is thus worse in males. Some of the secretions of the ovary and the adrenals in women, however, also contribute to acne.

The first stage of acne, that of the "blackhead," is caused by accumulation of secretion in the little duct of an oil gland which may have become plugged up. Chemical changes in the secretion turn it dark, resulting in the blackhead itself. Enlargement and inflammation of the oil gland may then occur, resulting in pimple formation. A variety of other factors may increase or decrease the severity of this process. Lack of sunshine, poor general health, the imminence of menstruation —perhaps also emotional stress—may aggravate acne; so, too, will an excess of certain food items, such as chocolate, nuts, candy, and fatty foods (and perhaps also food items rich in iodide, such as shellfish). Secondary infection by some of the bacteria that are generally present on the skin, notably the staphylococcal organisms, will aggravate the process.

Most cases of acne leave no scarring; with more severe forms, healing results in the formation of "pits." Even in the absence of scarring, many teenagers find acne a distressing disorder which increases their doubts about their appearance and makes them feel unhappily conspicuous; this condition should therefore not be dismissed as a passing growth-event. A normal teenager interested in appearance will appreciate parental and medical attention directed to acne.

Treatment. Although acne is treated in different ways by various doctors, the following are generally useful hints:

1. Soap-and-water cleanliness is important. The face should be washed several times daily. One of the newer germ-killing soaps may be helpful in keeping down the element of infection.

2. A cotton pledget soaked in rubbing alcohol may be wiped across the forehead, nose, or other oily and broken-out areas several times daily. Prepackaged pledgets moistened with alcohol are available in tinfoil and are easily carried about.

3. Lotions and creams which cut down the activity of the oil glands can be applied one or more times daily as directed; most contain sulphur, salicylic acid, and similar ingredients, and have a drying and peeling effect.

4. Sunlight—to the point of slight tanning and burning— is good for acne. The acne patient should get plenty of sun

in the summertime and might well take ultraviolet lamp treatments throughout the winter.

5. Where pus formation and the element of infection seem important, antibiotics may be prescribed.

▶ **Acne Rosacea** This is a skin disorder, predominantly of the face, which bears some resemblance to ordinary acne. It is, however, more common in women, particularly past the age of thirty, and especially in those with a lifelong tendency to easy blushing. Redness of the skin is an almost constant finding, usually associated with oiliness, enlargement of the oil glands, and pustule formation; it is made worse by sunlight, hot beverages, alcoholic drinks, and emotional tension. It has been found that many patients with acne rosacea lead psychologically stressful lives and have difficulty in relaxing. The nose, which is most often the first area involved, usually shows some degree of redness much of the time; later the forehead, cheeks, and chin tend to show involvement. The tiny blood vessels of the skin become more prominent, and this may persist even after treatment.

Treatment. Treatment somewhat resembles that for acne, except that sun should be avoided, along with extremes of weather and hot or alcoholic beverages. Sulphur ointment is useful when applied to the skin, and frequent washing with soap and water is desirable. Learning a "take-it-easy" attitude may well be made part of the treatment.

▶ **Athlete's Foot** This is a common fungus infection of the feet, often chronic, and difficult to eradicate because of the hardiness of the organism responsible for it. In most instances it is more of a minor nuisance than a major skin disorder. However, a relatively mild form may spread in hot weather with great rapidity. Minor forms are found in the skin between the toes, most commonly between the third, fourth, and fifth toes and seldom involving the big toe. The skin has a soggy or opaque appearance, or may appear thinner than usual and be reddened. Oozing and cracking can occur and produce itching and pain. Occasionally the eruption spreads over the sole of the foot and produces patches of redness, swelling, and moisture. Sometimes infection with other organisms occurs; increased swelling, and pain and pus formation, may follow. However, in another form of the disease the eruption is dry and scaly. In certain sensitive individuals an eruption—known

265

as the "id" reaction—which resembles tiny blisters may appear on the palms and fingers. This is not an actual infection of the skin of the hands but is rather an allergic reaction to some substance produced by the fungi in the feet; the id eruption clears up when the fungus infection of the feet is brought under control.

Treatment. Treatment of athlete's foot will depend upon the extent and kind of infection present. For an acute, spreading, weeping, or secondarily-infected eruption the patient may have to get off his feet for a time. Soaking in potassium permanganate solution or Burow's solution may be useful at this stage. Once this acute stage is controlled, the usual measures can be employed. These include the following:

1. Applying Whitfield's ointment.
2. Applying solutions and ointments containing fatty acids.
3. Washing feet daily with a bacteria-killing soap.
4. Wearing open-toed shoes or sandals, with as much exposure of the feet as possible. The organism cannot grow on a dry foot.
5. Wearing cotton hose since they are more absorptive than synthetic or wool.
6. Continuing the powders and ointments even after the condition seems to have cleared, since athlete's foot is notorious for recurring.

▶ **Dandruff** Dandruff, referred to by doctors as seborrheic dermatitis, can vary from a little flakiness deposited on the hair and clothing to larger, reddened or crusty patches on the scalp. It is considered a disturbance of the oil glands of the scalp; it is not uncommonly found together with acne or with seborrheic dermatitis of the chest and face—all of which involve some disordered function of the oil-making (sebaceous) glands. Most cases of dandruff are mild and need not cause concern, for they do not worsen with the passage of time. Sometimes if a shampooing is skipped, particularly if the hair grows thickly, some itching may occur. This may also be aggravated by oily or greasy hairdressings and by hair-styling which plasters the hair down and prevents airing of the scalp.

Milder cases of dandruff can be kept under control simply by shampooing once or twice a week. Tincture of green soap, available at the drugstore counter, may be more efficacious than ordinary soap. In addition there are various prepared shampoos specifically designed to be of aid in dandruff control. Many of these can be bought over the counter, but other effective ones are available on the doctor's prescription.

▶ **Eczema** Eczema is an allergic skin disorder characterized by itching, scaling, and oozing lesions. (In urticaria, a less severe form, hives appear which are raised red wheals of either small or giant size; these are extremely itchy.) The itching causes scratching which in turn produces bleeding; frequently secondary infection appears. In infants, eczema usually appears first on the face, the cheeks, and the creases and folds of the arms and legs. Eczema may be caused by sensitivity to milk, eggs, wool, soaps, oils, etc.

Treatment. Treatment of eczema is directed toward removing the offending allergen and applying soothing lotions and ointments to the skin in order to heal it. Wet, oozing types of eczema can be treated with Burow's solution compresses, or with soaking in potassium permanganate. More severe cases require medication such as cortisone and cortisone-containing ointments. Treatment can also be accomplished by desensitization with specific antigens.

▶ **Impetigo Contagiosa** This is a contagious disease of the skin characterized by pustules and crusts. The crusted type is caused by *streptococcus pyogenes;* the bulbous type is caused by *staphylococcus pyogenes.* It is a common secondary invader of any irritation or rash. It appears most commonly on the face, hands, neck, ears, and upper and lower extremities. It starts as a pimple which becomes a blister, filling with pus. Then the yellowish material drains out and produces a raw, wet, pustular surface. Impetigo is treated with antibiotics, both in ointment form and by injection.

▶ **Neurodermatitis** This is an often stubborn skin reaction which generally occurs in older children. It is characterized by itchy, dry, red, raised, scaly lesions which become thickened so that they appear lichenified. The most common areas for this rash are in the creases of the elbows, the back of the neck, and the creases behind the knees. Treatment is the same as for many allergic conditions of the skin.

▶ **Psoriasis** This is a common chronic skin disorder which tends to run in some family groupings. A major feature of the disorder is scale formation; the scales are white, are often shed

267

in large numbers, and are most commonly found over the knees, elbows, and the scalp. There is seldom any itching. Although psoriasis can occur at any age, it is not common before the age of four. Various general infections and menstruation make psoriasis worse; pregnancy often improves it. Small localized forms of the disease can be left alone. More extensive forms may be discouragingly conspicuous. It is important to recognize that, although psoriasis is chronic, it can be helped and the lesions may stay cleared for many months after successful treatment.

Treatment. Sunlight often helps psoriasis, this being the basis for the approach known as the Goekerman treatment. In this, a coal tar ointment is applied to the area of psoriasis, and increasing doses of ultraviolet from an ultraviolet lamp are given daily. The ultraviolet exposure is built up in ordinary tanning treatments, by increasing the exposure slightly each day. After the treatment, the scales can be scrubbed away and more ointment rubbed into the area. Another form of treatment suitable when the disease is not too extensive involves application of a steroid (cortisone-type) ointment. The area is then covered with Saran® wrap. The Saran wrap may be left undisturbed for several days, and the treatment may be repeated as directed by the physician. Sometimes dietary approaches, such as low-protein intake, may be tried.

▶ **Ringworm (Tinea Circinata)** Ringworm of the skin is a contagious fungus disease, showing a circular lesion with a raised border. It may be contracted from animals, household pets or from direct contact with infected persons. It appears first as a small pink-to-reddish round patch (the size of a small pea to that of a quarter), with some scaliness in the center. It is very itchy. Treatment is by the proper use of fungicidal remedies. Tincture of iodine, sulfur, ammoniated mercury, and other drugs have been used with success.

▶ **Scabies** This is a highly contagious itching rash which consists of little papules, vesicles (blisters), and crusts resulting from secondary infection and scratching. It is caused by an organism, *Sarcoptes scabiei* (mite), also called the "itch mite." Usually, if one member of a family has this condition, others become infected. It is frequently seen as a wavy line on the palms of the hands, the soles of the feet, or on other areas of the body. The itching usually occurs at night. It is generally necessary for a physician to make the diagnosis; he can then prescribe the proper medication to clear up the condition.

▶ **Urticaria (Hives) and Angioneurotic Edema** Hives are small, red, raised lesions of the skin which break out and cause severe itching. They may appear in single pimples or in clusters and may be large in diameter or very tiny.

Giant hives are characterized by very large areas of swelling (edema) which may appear in any part of the skin or mucous membranes. There may be swelling and puffiness of the eyes and lids, and puffiness of the throat in which there may be a sensation of choking. The skin may become red and itchy. The causes are generally the same as those of hives, that is, some specific allergen or possibly a psychological cause. The treatment is the same as for other allergies.

SKIN CONDITIONS IN INFANTS

▶ **Cradle Cap (Seborrheic Dermatitis)** This is a condition in infants characterized by thick yellow-brown crusts on the scalp. It occasionally appears on the brows and behind the ears. It is often due to inadequate cleansing of the scalp.

Bland oils (olive oil, sweet almond oil, petrolatum, etc.) are used to soften the crusts. Then the hair can be washed and the crusts fine-combed out. If this home treatment does not effectively clear the scalp, consult your doctor.

▶ **Diaper Rash (Ammonia Dermatitis)** This is a rash characterized by red, raised pimples and flat areas around the surfaces of the thighs, buttocks, and frequently on the lower half of the abdomen. There is usually a strong odor of ammonia present in the diapers.

The treatment of this condition, first of all, is to remove the wet diaper as soon as possible, so that it does not remain in contact with the tender skin. Use of ointments or powders to prevent bacterial decomposition in this area will help. There are also pills, to be given by mouth, which metabolize the ammonia in the urine to its less toxic product and prevent its further formation. Severe diaper rash may go on to secondary infection and require use of antibiotics. Special superabsorbent diaper liners are also helpful in reducing rash.

▶ **Intertrigo** This is a chafing from the effects of heat and moisture, and is seen in the creases of the skin, particularly in fat babies. It usually occurs in the groin, neck and underneath the armpits. Proper cleansing and proper washing of the skin, as well as changing soiled diapers frequently, is important in the prevention of this condition.

▶ **Perianal Dermatitis** This is an area of redness, inflammation, and rash localized around the anus and rectal area. Its cause is not known, but sometimes the stool and its chemicals produce it by irritating the skin around the rectum. It may be confused with typical "diaper rash," which usually has a strong ammonia odor associated with it. In perianal dermatitis there is usually no odor of ammonia.

Proper cleansing of the perianal region by using cotton moistened with warm water or vaseline, with care to remove all the stool from the area, is important. It may be necessary to leave the diaper off and expose the child to a 100-watt bulb, placed about 18 inches above the buttocks. This will dry the rash and help to clear it.

▶ **Prickly Heat (Miliaria)** This is caused by overheating and excessive clothing. Approximately 75 to 80 per cent of body heat loss occurs through the skin by evaporation or perspiration. Prickly heat occurs during the hot summer days and is characterized by tiny, red, raised pimples all over the skin. Witch hazel water is an excellent evaporating lotion for the prevention and treatment of this condition. It may be patted on the skin daily, and followed by dusting with ordinary cornstarch or an unscented talc. Bathing in starch or bicarbonate of soda is helpful in overcoming skin irritation.

▶ **Roseola Infantum** Contagious.

Cause. Virus.

Incubation period. 1 to 2 weeks.

Symptoms. Convulsions frequently usher in roseola with high fever up to 105° and 106°F. There is little to account for the sudden onset and marked irritability in these infants except, sometimes, a slight sore throat. The fever remains high and fluctuating for three or four days. Then it suddenly drops and a rash breaks out, usually on the trunk, subsequently spreading to the arms and neck, occasionally on the face. The rash is light pink, flat, approximately the size of small split peas. It fades within twenty-four to forty-eight hours.

There is no treatment necessary because by the time the rash breaks out and the disease is recognized, it is over. Roseola resembles regular measles, allergic drug rashes, and German measles. It is usually necessary for a doctor to distinguish which condition is present.

SMALLPOX (VARIOLA)   Contagious.

Cause. Virus.

Incubation period. Usually 12 to 14 days, but may be as long as 16 to 21 days.

Symptoms. The disease is transmitted by droplet infection via the respiratory tract. There is usually a long period of mild symptoms, such as fever, headache, malaise, and back pain, before the rash breaks out. A slight rash, which resembles measles or scarlet fever, may appear during the first two days. Then it becomes raised and pustular and begins to look exactly like smallpox vaccinations. These are first distributed mainly on arms and legs, then travel toward the trunk and body. They tend to be deeper and the centers are depressed. Whereas in chicken pox there are different stages of the rash present at the same time, in smallpox they are all more or less at the same stage at each phase of the disease.

Prevention. Vaccination with the virus of cow pox is performed on the skin during the first year of life. In three or four days a pimple forms which becomes a blister, then fills with pus. There may be a red ring around the vaccination about the size of a dime or quarter. After five to seven days a fever may develop, and the child may become irritable and fretful. The scab which forms on the vaccination should be protected with a bandage until it falls off spontaneously; otherwise it may leave a deep, pitted scar. If the vaccination does not "take" the first time, it should be repeated after a few months. It is extremely dangerous to vaccinate a child who has any open sores, allergic rashes, or eczema until the rash is cleared completely. Nor should vaccine be administered to a child in whose family any of the above skin rashes exist (unless the others have already been vaccinated). Open skin lesions will attract the virus and start a case flaring with scattered smallpox lesions. This condition, in a child who has eczema, is called "eczema vaccinatum" and will leave serious skin scars.

SMOKING   The only form of smoking that has been particularly singled out as a health hazard is the smoking of cigarettes. The risks associated with smoking pipes and cigars are markedly less. The case against cigarettes has been building up for many years and was given impressive endorsement by the Surgeon General's Report in 1964; however, as early as 1938 it had been demonstrated that heavy smokers, on average, lived four years less than non-smokers. Cigarette smoking unquestionably contributes to a great many major lung diseases, ranging from lung cancer to chronic bronchitis and a condition known as emphysema which produces breathlessness on effort. There is some evidence that it also increases the work of the heart and that the incidence of heart attacks is higher in smokers. The major problem is not with establishing the truth of the accusations, but rather with the difficulty cigarette smokers encounter in giving up the habit. A lucky few find it can be given up with ease; the majority find it difficult and trying. Nevertheless, medical men who best know the facts deplore the willingness of smokers to run the risks involved.

Surveys indicate that the highest percentage of ex-smokers is to be found among doctors. If men who know tobacco best have quit—why shouldn't you? Insofar as pregnancy is concerned, there is no evidence that cigarette smoking has any significant effect on the development of the child. Some evidence does indicate that the child may be slightly smaller in cigarette-smoking mothers, but the difference is not very significant. However, our knowledge about tobacco is only a recently acquired one and is still undergoing change.

Since no one pretends to know it all, it might not be considered unreasonable to include tobacco in a general ban against all drugs—except the necessary ones—during pregnancy. Since the nausea often experienced in early pregnancy tends to do away with the desire to smoke anyway, giving up cigarettes for the duration, if not longer, may be a relatively easier step at that time. Certainly heavy smoking, one or two packs a day or more, is best drastically cut down. Statistics indicate that all of the difficulties produced by tobacco increase considerably above the ten-cigarette per day limit.

SPINAL COLUMN   The spinal column consists of a series of vertebrae which extend from the skull down to a terminal portion. The latter can be felt adjacent to the rectal region and is known as the coccyx or tailbone. The vertebrae are sometimes referred to in terms of their location: the cervical vertebrae, of which there are seven, form the neck region; the twelve thoracic vertebrae have ribs extending from them and form the main bony support to the trunk; the five lumbar vertebrae form the small of the back. These twenty-four vertebrae are capable of movement. Below them are the five sacral segments which contribute to the posterior aspect of the pelvis, and below those, the four little segments which make up the coccyx. The sacral and coccygeal segments are sometimes referred to as false or fixed vertebrae, and lack motion.

Between the true vertebrae there are fibrous disks with a central more gelatinous portion called the *nucleus pulposus.* Occasionally the nucleus pulposus works loose from its central location and impinges on one of the spinal nerves. This produces a radiating type of neuritis which may be quite severe and is sometimes referred to as a radiculitis; it is a common cause of sciatica. Between the vertebrae are openings for the spinal nerves, called the intervertebral foramina. Occasionally bony spurs that form because of osteoarthritis can produce pressure on the emerging nerves—another form of neuritis.

▶ **Disorders of the Spinal Column** The infant has a backbone which is a single long curve from the head down to the buttocks. As the child grows and assumes the upright position, a series of curves normally appears in the vertebral column. This produces two hollows, one in the neck, the other in the small of the back, plus two outward bowings, one in the trunk and the other in the sacral region. It is thought that the curve in the lumbosacral region is one of the anatomical "facts of life" which leads to the frequency of backache in human beings; it can be regarded as one of the penalties for assuming our erect position.

Curvature of the spine to one side or the other is most often seen in the thoracic region and produces a condition known as scoliosis. Unequal rates of growth in the centers which lay down the bone of the vertebrae can lead to scoliosis. There is also a hereditary background, for it may be seen in more than one member of a family. Mild degrees of this disorder can be disregarded, but in other instances the curvature may be progressive. This can lead to various types of chest deformities. There are usually associated pains in the chest and there may be interference with lung function. Various orthopedic procedures for correcting scoliosis are available.

Since the vertebrae encase the spinal cord, injuries to them pose a special threat. Cord damage can produce symptoms varying from pain to weakness and on to paralysis. Hence the reason for caution in treating accident victims who may have a back injury. Some of the loss of height seen in elderly individuals, particularly women, is due to narrowing of the vertebrae. This is a condition known as osteoporosis—a loss of substance and calcium from bone. The vertebrae, being subject to the stress of weight bearing, may be among the first bones to give indication of this disorder. Various factors contribute to this condition, including inadequate calcium intakes over the years and the diminishing hormones after the change of life.

STEAM INHALATIONS, HOW TO PREPARE   Steam inhalations may be prescribed when children have croup, hoarseness, sore throat, or difficulty in breathing. Breathing a warm, moist mixture of air usually relieves the swelling in the tissues of the nose and throat and eases breathing. There are many good commercial vaporizers for sale. If you buy one, it is important to get the kind which will run automatically all night so that you do not have to get up every few hours to replace the water in it.

If you wish to make a homemade vaporizer, these are the things you will require: a hotplate with a teakettle, a long funnel which you can make out of newspapers or aluminum foil, an umbrella, and some sheets. The umbrella is used to make a canopy over the child's bed. The sheet is draped over the umbrella so that it makes a tent. This permits the steam to enter only the area in the child's bed and not dissipate itself in the rest of the room. A blanket may be used over the sheet. Since there will be a great deal of moisture, it may be well to wrap the child's head in a towel or scarf, so that the wet hair does not become uncomfortable.

The teakettle, with water in it, is placed on the hotplate on a stool or chair near the side of the bed. The funnel is directed so that the steam does not hit the child directly in the face, nor should it be close enough to cause a steam burn. It is very important to avoid scalding. The water can be kept boil-

274

ing as long as treatment is required. Fresh water may be added as needed. It is important to make sure that the kettle is not within reach of the child's hand. It is best to stay with him while the treatment is continuing.

STERILITY AND INFERTILITY   Sterility is said to exist in a woman when, despite normal sexual relations, she fails to become pregnant. A somewhat related condition consists of difficulty in becoming pregnant as often as is desired, as may occur when a couple has only one or two children although they attempt to have more. If no contraceptive methods are used, a young, sexually vigorous couple can anticipate that pregnancy will occur within a year, and it may, of course, occur quite a bit sooner. If it becomes clear with the passage of time that the marriage is a sterile one, a "sterility work-up" may be called for.

Since a sterile marriage can be due to the male rather than the female, and since the male partner's role is easy to evaluate, the husband may be checked first. After establishing that he is in good health and suffers no endocrine or other disease which might affect sexual performance, a semen examination will generally be the next step. By examining such a specimen the doctor can determine whether a normal number of sperm cells are being furnished, and whether these cells appear normal under the microscope.

The equivalent question to be answered in the case of the woman is whether or not she is ovulating, that is, whether an egg is being formed and released from the ovaries each month. There are various ways of establishing this, some simple, others complicated. One of the simplest is the daily temperature record. This involves taking the temperature with a specially designed thermometer the first thing in the morning before arising, and recording the temperature. In a normal cycle there is generally a slight temperature rise at about the middle of the cycle, corresponding to the time of ovulation. The temperature rise remains for the next two weeks, then rapidly declines with the onset of menstruation. Such a temperature change around mid-cycle is fairly good, though not conclusive, evidence of ovulation.

Sometimes a blockage of the tubes which run from the ovary to the uterus may be responsible for sterility. This can be determined by a tubal insufflation test. In this procedure air is blown up into the tubes and the pressure recorded by a measuring device. An X-ray can be taken simultaneously. The test will reveal whether or not a blockage of the tubes is present. Other tests that may be performed include analysis of the urine for its hormone content, which may also give evidence for ovulation, and biopsies.

Both general and specific measures are often indicated in cases of infertility. Moderate to marked degrees of overweight in women may be associated with menstrual irregularity and lack of fertility, so that a reducing program may be advised. Some doctors almost routinely give some of their patients thyroid by mouth, on the theory that its generally stimulating value may be of use. It is often advised that sexual relations be restricted to the time of ovulation, or at least more frequently indulged in then. It is also sometimes advised that women lie on their backs with their legs drawn up for perhaps a half hour after intercourse. Occasionally plastic operations on the tubes if there is evidence of blockage, or for repositioning a uterus that is very markedly tipped backwards, are advised. In the rare instances where failure to form eggs in the ovary is the cause for sterility, with the tubes and everything else seemingly normal, hormone preparations designed to produce ovulation have been experimented with successfully.

SUNBURN   The sun's rays are capable of producing injury to the skin quite comparable to that produced by a flame. One of the chief differences is that in sunburn the extent of the injury may be seen only after some hours, and its development is gradual. In addition to marked reddening and burning sensations, blistering may occur. When a considerable skin area is involved, the individual may feel sick and have chilly sensations, weakness, and perhaps also headache and some fever.

In most instances sunburn is due to an overenthusiastic attempt to become tanned too rapidly. It sometimes results from falling asleep while out in the sun, something that is often avoidable. Blondes and redheads are generally more susceptible than brunettes, and infants and children are more susceptible than adults. Certain drugs, as some of the sulfonamides, may also sensitize the skin to the sun. Remember, too, that pregnancy also increases susceptibility to sunburning.

A brunette should probably have no more than one or two fifteen-minute exposures at the first sunning. As pigmentation develops, skin tolerance increases and the periods of exposure can be lengthened. Blondes and others with sensitive skins should probably get no more than five minutes of sun under the same circumstances. Reflections from sand, water, and ice increase the intensity of the exposure time. Numerous commercial preparations are available for screening out the skin-damaging components of sunshine while permitting tanning to occur.

Mild cases of sunburn are often disregarded; the discomfort can be somewhat relieved by powders containing zinc oxide and zinc stearate, or by local dabbing with calamine lotion or with cold cream. Where there has been some blistering, oatmeal or starch baths will be soothing. A starch bath is prepared by mixing two cups of cornstarch with water to form a paste and adding it to a tub bath. After soaking in this, the individual may allow the starch to dry on the skin. Aspirin and other pain-diminishing drugs may be used for the burning pain. Steroids are sometimes prescribed to diminish the reaction in the skin. Peeling of the skin and tanning are the usual consequences of a sunburn, and these may be more marked in a pregnant woman. For a severe sunburn, especially if there is any sign of infection in the blisters, a doctor should be consulted.

SUPPOSITORIES   Suppositories are specially designed and molded solids which are inserted into a bodily orifice. Their composition is such that they melt at body temperature and release their medicinal agents. Rectal and vaginal suppositories are by far the most common. Occasionally, a suppository destined to be introduced into the urethra, the urinary channel, may be prescribed. Many suppositories have a cocoa-butter base or other ingredients which soften at room temperature, particularly on hot days. This may make them more difficult to insert, in which case they are probably best kept in the refrigerator.

Hemorrhoidal suppositories generally contain a mixture of medicines designed to promote healing in combination with a local anesthetic which will relieve some of the pain or discomfort. When both external and internal hemorrhoids are present, the external ones may be lightly coated by rubbing them with the suppository before insertion. The familiar glycerine suppository, generally dispensed in adult and child sizes, releases glycerine as it melts. This produces a local irritant effect and initiates a desire to move the bowels. More recent suppositories for the same purpose contain agents which stimulate the bowel musculature and may produce a movement within five to ten minutes. A variety of drugs are available in suppository form. They are particularly useful when nausea or vomiting occur.

Vaginal suppositories are widely used, particularly for the treatment of infections such as trichomoniasis and moniliasis. Vaginal suppositories contain such varied agents as antibiotics, organic compounds of arsenic, synthetic organic compounds, and even so simple an agent as lactose, a sugar which in the course of its breakdown will raise the vaginal acidity.

TEETH   The milk teeth, or temporary teeth (deciduous) are all erupted by two and a half years of age. There are twenty of them. They appear in approximately the following order:

  6 to 8 months—2 lower central incisors
  8 to 12 months—4 upper incisors
                   2 lower lateral incisors
  12 to 16 months—4 anterior molars
  16 to 20 months—4 canines
  12 to 30 months—4 posterior molars

In order to determine approximately how many temporary teeth should be present in your child, subtract six from the age of the child in months. That is, at ten months your child should have approximately four teeth.

There are thirty-two permanent teeth. These appear in approximately the following order:

  6 years of age—4 first molars
  7 to 9 years of age—8 incisors
  10 to 12 years—8 bicuspids
  11 to 12 years— 4 canines
  13 years—4 second molars
  17 to 22 years—4 third molars

Salivation begins at about three or four months of age. In most instances, infants drool and do not swallow the saliva.

This usually indicates that teething will begin shortly. Many infants become slightly irritable and fussy, with occasional low fevers and insomnia, during the period preceding the eruption of teeth. The temperature usually does not go above 100° or 100.5°F. The gums may be painful and sore, and there are many medications which can be rubbed on them to relieve the pain. In addition, aspirin and teething rings may be used. If fever persists, call your doctor.

▶ **Fluorides** Fluorides retard the development of cavities in the teeth of children, hence some communities have fluoridated their water supplies. If your water supply is fluoridated, it will not be necessary to give your child supplementary fluorides in his vitamins. However, there is considerable controversy regarding the safety of administering fluorides, which have been the subject of many large-scale studies and series for years. If your child should develop mottling, or speckling of the teeth, it may be an indication that fluorides should be stopped.

TEETH, CARE OF Children can be taught to brush their own teeth from about the age of two. It has recently been shown that children who from infancy drink water containing minute quantities of fluorine do not develop as many cavities as those who do not. If your community does not have fluoridated water, it may be desirable to add fluoride to your child's diet in the form of fluoridated vitamins.

Regular visits to the dentist will help in maintaining healthy teeth. Healthy teeth are important for general good health. They make us more attractive, help us speak well, and help us digest food by chewing it properly. Good nutrition with all the essential food elements is necessary to develop and maintain healthy teeth and gums. When food particles are left between the teeth, bacteria in the mouth produce acids that dissolve the enamel and form cavities. It is, therefore, advisable, to brush teeth after eating in order to remove trapped food.

Brushing should be performed away from the gums instead of toward them so that food will not be pushed under the gum margins. Separate toothbrushes should belong to each member of the family and not be used interchangeably.

▶ **Pyorrhea (Periodontitis)** This is a condition that attacks the tissues around the teeth. It causes the tooth sockets to become loose, and finally the teeth either fall out or must be removed. The infection begins with an inflammation of the gums called gingivitis. The gums bleed easily and food wedges in the spaces between the teeth. If there is also malocclusion (upper and lower teeth which do not fit together), it may contribute to infections of the gum. In cases where the upper and lower teeth do not fit together properly, a dentist may decide that braces or other treatment may be necessary to get them into proper alignment.

TEETH—MALOCCLUSION Malocclusion refers to departures from the normal in the way in which the teeth meet. As with many other facial features, hereditary factors may play a part. Thus, one may see "buckteeth" and other disorders in several members of one family. Because the genes determining the size of the upper and lower jaw may be inherited separately from the two parents, a structural disharmony with malocclusion may result.

Too early loss of baby teeth may allow a shifting from the normal position of some of the permanent teeth. In fact, even in the adult, loss of teeth frequently leads to shifts in the position of adjacent teeth, and production of an acquired malocclusion. In the young child, such a shift is sometimes prevented by placing a device between the remaining teeth so that they will not move together and crowd a tooth that is still to come; such a device is referred to as a "space saver." Other causes for malocclusion are: failure of certain teeth to erupt; eruption of teeth in such a manner that significant spaces exist; or out-of-line eruption of teeth.

Much of the loss of teeth experienced by middle-aged individuals is not due to dental decay but to bad bite. As a result of bad bite, there is a resorption of bone around the sockets, with loosening of the teeth. This can lead to their ultimate loss.

Malocclusion also increases the incidence of dental decay; hence most dentists believe that correction of most malocclusions is well worth the time, effort, and expense. Usually wires or molds are used to slowly push some of the teeth into a more desirable location. In order to do this and achieve a good bite, several teeth may sometimes have to be pulled—as in those instances where the jaw is small and the teeth are crowded. Children wearing the various braces and bands that are necessary may be somewhat more subject to dental decay. They should accordingly be cautioned against eating candy or sweet and sticky foods, drinking carbonated beverages, and chewing gum.

TEMPERATURE, TAKING   Temperature indicates the heat of the body. It may be taken in many areas of the body. In infants and children the rectal area is the one generally accepted since it determines the internal temperature of the body most readily. Small children should not be permitted to hold a glass thermometer in the mouth. They will often bite it off or permit it to drop and break.

There are two types of thermometers—rectal and oral. The rectal thermometer has a blunt, short bulb containing the mercury. The oral thermometer has a long thin bulb. A thermometer should be held at the end opposite to the mercury. It should never be placed or cleansed in hot water, since this would shoot the mercury up past the level at which the temperature is calibrated and break the thermometer. Normal temperature is about 98.6° to 99.4°F. with fluctuations of 0.2 to 0.6 degrees. It may sometimes be as low as 97°F.

To take a child's temperature, the child should be placed on one's lap, lying prone or on his back, and the thermometer lubricated with vaseline (or some other lubricant) and inserted about one-third to halfway into the rectum. It is held there for about two to three minutes, removed, and cleansed with a piece of alcohol-soaked cotton. The temperature is read and recorded, then the thermometer is shaken down with a snapping motion of the wrist. This reduces the mercury to below the normal level. If this is not done, then when one takes the temperature again it will show a recording at a higher-than-normal level.

Temperature taken by mouth may be slightly lower than that taken by rectum. Sometimes there is as much as one degree of difference.

Temperature can be taken under the armpits or in the groin by placing the thermometer in one of these areas, with instructions to keep the arm or leg close to the body. It may be necessary to keep the thermometer in this position for five to seven minutes in order to get an accurate reading. Temperature should be taken every three or four hours, and if the fever is high, every hour. (See also FEVER.)

TETANUS (LOCKJAW)   Contagious.

Cause. Bacterial, *Clostridium tetani.*

Incubation period. 1 to 3 weeks.

The infection is via a contaminated wound. The organism which causes this disease is widely distributed in the soil in many parts of the world. Under certain conditions, it gets into the skin and bloodstream and produces several poisons. One of these destroys red blood cells, another injures white blood cells and produces a poison which causes the muscle rigidity and spasm for which this disease is noted. There is no suitable skin test to determine immunity. Any type of wound may give rise to tetanus if the germs enter that area. Any injury or skin cut which has been contaminated by dirt should therefore be carefully cleansed and treated, and immunization given to prevent tetanus. Tetanus is also popularly known as "lockjaw." The reason for this name is that during the onset, which is gradual, there is increasing spasm of the neck and jaw muscles (trismus) with difficulty in swallowing and opening the mouth.

Symptoms. They include irritability, fever, chills, pains, headaches, convulsions, and coma. The spasm is quite characteristic in which the body is rigid as a board. The head is drawn back with the legs and feet extended. The arms are stiff and the hands clenched. The spasm of the facial muscles results in a fixed expression which looks like a sardonic grin.

Treatment. Tetanus is a very serious disease. The mortality rate, even with treatment, is about 50 per cent. Immediate hospitalization is necessary and tetanus antitoxin plus sedatives are required. It is extremely important to prevent choking. Antibiotics and antitoxin are usually used.

Prevention. Tetanus toxoid injections, either singly or in triple toxoid form, followed by booster injections, should be started during the first year of life.

THUMB-SUCKING   Sucking is a reflex activity in newborn infants. Stroking the lips produces sucking as soon as the infant is given a nipple. It is one of the child's first pleas-

282

ures and satisfactions. Unless adequate sucking is given to children, many develop unsatisfied "oral" needs in later life. This may be seen in overeating, smoking, chewing, and other oral excesses. Some babies finish the bottle rapidly, not really getting enough sucking. They may continue to suck on their thumbs or fingers because it is pleasurable. Pacifiers are sucked instead of fingers by some infants.

Sucking needs usually diminish after the children are able to drink from a cup or glass, but many of them continue to suck their thumbs for years afterwards. This persistence of immature gratification may be an indication of unsatisfied emotional needs, inadequate attention to the child so that he has to look to himself for gratification; or it may be a habit which the parents have never really taken the trouble to discourage. If thumb-sucking persists into later years, and there is pushing of the dental arch, disorders of the teeth and gums may occur. Parents can often divert young children from sucking their fingers by playing with them and keeping them occupied in other ways.

Most cases of finger- or thumb-sucking are outgrown after the age of two or so, when the child is able to move about on his own and is not entirely dependent upon parents for the satisfaction of needs. Most children who feel a firm family affection and receive sufficient attention do not need to resort to thumb-sucking for their own emotional satisfaction. If sucking persists into older years, psychological treatment may be necessary.

THYROID GLAND DISORDERS

▶ **Goiter** Enlargement of the thyroid gland is termed goiter. The gland is located in the lower portion of the neck, with its two main lobes on either side of the trachea or windpipe. Hence any significant goiter may be readily visible on inspection of the neck, particularly if the head is thrown backwards. Various terms are used by doctors to classify thyroid enlargements.

A toxic goiter is one producing excessive amounts of thyroid hormone; the associated symptoms are nervousness, tremor, rapid pulse, weight loss, crying spells. A non-toxic goiter is one that does not produce excess thyroid hormone. A diffuse goiter is one in which the enlargement occurs quite equally throughout the entire gland. A nodular goiter is one in which generally small nodules or lumps are felt scattered throughout the thyroid substance.

Sometimes the cause or a significant symptom is referred to, as in iodine-deficiency goiter, in which lack of iodine in the diet produces the enlargement; or exophthalmic goiter, a common form of goiter associated with prominent, "staring" appearance of the eyes. Virtually all enlargements of the thyroid are benign, but occasionally one is not, and may be referred to as a malignant goiter. Even so, many cancers of the thyroid are classified as low-grade tumors with little propensity to spread, and curiously enough, some may be controlled by thyroid administration.

Treatment. Treatment of a goiter is dependent upon its type. A toxic goiter may be treated by surgery, radioactive iodine, or certain antithyroid drugs. Some forms of goiter respond well to the administration of thyroid by mouth, and in iodine-deficiency goiter some form of iodine or iodized salt may be prescribed. Minor degrees of enlargement may remain untreated. The thyroid gland is normally slightly larger in women than in men, and may undergo some further enlargement in pregnancy. This represents an enlargement compatible with the need for increased output. No special measures are indicated for this sort of size increase.

▶ **Hyperthyroidism** Overactivity of the thyroid gland leads to the condition known as *hyperthyroidism*. Common complaints here are loss of weight, a ravenous appetite, sensations of great warmth, tremors, nervousness, palpitations and other disorders of the heart, and sometimes diarrhea. This condition is usually associated with an obvious enlargement of the thyroid gland, and—particularly in younger individuals—prominence of the eyes. Some of the diagnostic aids used to determine the degree of hyperthyroidism include: (1) The basal metabolism test, a test of the amount of oxygen consumed; this rises in hyperthyroidism. (2) The protein-bound iodine (PBI) test. In this, determination is made of the amounts of thyroid hormone circulating in the blood. (3) The radioactive iodine uptake test. In this, a minute amount of radioactive iodine is taken as a drink—the "atomic cocktail." Next, measurements are made over the thyroid gland to determine the amount of iodine that has been picked up there. In overactivity of the thyroid, more than twice the normal amount may be taken up.

▶ **Hypothyroidism** Underfunctioning of the thyroid gland, called *hypothyroidism* and sometimes referred to as "sluggish thyroid," is seen most often in women in their middle years. The condition develops slowly and stealthily, so that it is difficult for the patient herself to fix the time of onset. The complaints are usually of a progressive degree of weakness, fatigability, sensitivity to cold, dryness of the skin and hair, menstrual changes, constipation. The hair may become thin, the skin dry and yellowish, the voice low and cracked, thinking and the emotions slowed down and blunted. Widespread disorders of so many organs point up the fact that thyroid hormone acts on all body cells. Hypothyroidism is easily corrected by taking thyroid hormone by mouth.

▶ **Thyroiditis** Thyroiditis refers to various forms of inflammation in the thyroid gland. Some have been observed in relation to respiratory illnesses and are thought to be of viral origin. In most forms of thyroiditis, however, no organisms can be found. Acute thyroiditis may begin with an obvious swelling in the thyroid gland, with pain and tenderness, and even with mild symptoms of hyperthyroidism due to excessive release of the hormone. The condition is generally treated with steroid drugs. Chronic forms of thyroiditis—in which the process goes on at a slow rate for months and for years—also occur, though they are rare. An obvious goiter may be formed. Treatment varies but may consist of thyroid hormone, steroid drugs, and occasionally surgery.

TOILET TRAINING   Successful toilet training is a complex procedure for the young child. All normal children accomplish this eventually, and it is therefore simply a matter of time before the process is completely mastered. Hence it is wise to be patient and wait until the child is sufficiently mature to master this procedure.

Voluntary and involuntary nerve impulses maintain control of the urine and bowels. In the early weeks and months of life, the muscles which guard the opening for the passage of waste materials remain contracted until a certain "fullness" is obtained which stimulates the relaxation of the sphincter muscle control. The amount of stimuli and the time vary in different infants. Some voluntary activity as the infant strains and squeezes may operate very early in life. Sometimes it is a difficult process for a small infant in a lying-down position to expel the stool by himself. It may be helpful to sit him in a propped-up position as he strains so that the force or effect of gravity will help.

Children usually wish to gain approval; until your child is able to cooperate when you let him know you want him to use the toilet, he may not be able to meet your demands. Keeping a child on the toilet for long periods, expressing anger, disapproval, and shame, will only confuse him and make him resentful. It may lead to a bitter struggle. It is not possible to force a child to learn to control his bowels without serious trauma to the personality.

Occasional accidents and lapses may occur after a child is completely trained, and certain situations of stress may be responsible for lapses in ability to hold urine and stool. Attitudes which shame or humiliate the child will only delay and impair training. This may leave character traits of a most undesirable nature. Punishments, scoldings, spankings, threats are usually useless, and may be harmful. An attitude of encouragement, reassurance, tolerance, and praise are the best approaches to encourage toilet training.

TONSILS AND ADENOIDS

▶ **Tonsils** The tonsils are two groups of lymphoid tissue located on each side of the back of the throat. Tonsils (and the adenoids which are located near them) are frequently the source of chronic and recurrent upper respiratory infections in children. Some children are particularly susceptible to tonsil infections. Frequently the infection extends into the ear. There is usually fever which can go as high as 104°, a sensation of sore throat, inability to swallow, lack of appetite, nasal obstruction, and possibly impaired hearing.

Many mild cases of tonsillitis will clear by themselves without the use of antibiotics. Aspirin may be helpful in reducing the pain and fever. However, many cases require the use of penicillin and other antibiotics. Most cases clear within seven to ten days. In other cases tonsillectomy may be required.

The indications for tonsillectomy in children are: chronic tonsillitis attacks with adenoidal and ear complications; extreme cases of mouth breathing due to enlarged and obstructive adenoids; and peritonsillar abscess with chronic draining glands. Children who have repeated attacks of tonsillitis accompanied by rheumatic fever or other complications should be considered for tonsillectomy. Massive tonsils which cause obstruction in eating and difficulties in speech and phonation should be removed. Except in unusual cases, it is advisable for the child to be at least four or five years old before tonsils are removed.

▶ **Adenoids** These are masses of lymphoid tissue located on the posterior throat wall and roof of the mouth, in the area above the tonsils. They commonly enlarge and block the nasopharynx, causing mouth-breathing, running nose, and snoring.

Chronic adenoiditis may cause a nasal or "adenoidal" quality in the voice, offensive breath, and impairment of taste and smell. It has been known to alter the facial expression so much that the child appears dull or stupid. Cough, particularly at night, may occur. Deafness may sometimes be a complication if the eustachian tube (the tube leading from the ear to the throat) is blocked. Enlarged adenoids may be seen with the use of a pharyngeal mirror. The most effective treatment is surgical removal. This is usually done along with tonsillectomy.

TUBERCULOSIS   Contagious.

Cause. Bacterial, *Mycobacterium tuberculosis.*

Incubation period. Highly variable, up to years.

Symptoms. Tuberculosis may occur in any organ of the body and may frequently resemble other diseases. The diagnosis is made by recovering and growing the organism in a culture or examining a typical X-ray picture, particularly of the lungs. There are certain changes in tissues which are characteristic of this germ.

In children, *primary tuberculosis* refers to the first infection of an individual with the tubercle bacillus. The primary focus (Ghon tubercle) is usually in the lungs and is the original site of entry of the germ. This first lesion heals over and becomes calcified. It is seen on X-ray as an old but inactive lesion. Many people have initial, original infections of this sort which never spread.

Lung lesions in older people are generally larger, and the bacilli may travel to and colonize in the regional lymph glands.

Infection may spread to bones, kidney, brain, etc., and it is possible to have tuberculosis without many symptoms. Such lesions remain in a quiescent state, but may also break down in the future and spread.

Tuberculosis is classified according to the organ and form in which it occurs.

Since symptoms of this disease may continue obscure until the disease is well under way, diagnostic *tuberculin testing* is of great importance. There are patch tests and intradermal skin tests in different strengths. Further tests, such as X-rays, sputum cultures and spinal fluid examination, may be required to recover the tubercle bacilli and confirm the diagnosis.

Treatment. Tuberculosis is now considered curable as a result of the development of new drugs, which have been extremely successful in arresting early and even relatively advanced infections. More severe conditions may not be curable by drug treatment and may require prolonged hospitalization or surgical procedures. The drugs used are: INH (isonicotinic acid hydrazide), streptomycin, and PAS (para-aminosalicylic acid).

Prevention. Periodic chest X-rays and skin testing locate existing lesions and prevent spread by contacts. All contacts who show signs of disease should be treated. Exposure to known positive cases should be carefully avoided. Passive immunization to tuberculosis is available with BCG (bacillus Calmette-Guerin). This is a vaccine composed of bovine (cow) tubercle bacilli whose virulence has been modified by special procedures. Vaccination with this material produces a limited immunity to infection with tuberculosis. It is especially indicated for persons who live in areas with high tuberculosis rates and those who have intimate contact with arrested cases.

ULCER, PEPTIC   A peptic ulcer is a defect in the lining of the digestive tract, produced by a process of self-digestion and generally due to stomach secretions. The most common location for a peptic ulcer is in the top part of the small intestine, called the duodenum. Less common, but by no means infrequent, are peptic ulcers of the stomach lining, and least frequent are those found in the lower part of the esophagus, the tubelike structure running from the mouth to the stomach. Based on their location, therefore, peptic ulcers are sometimes referred to as *duodenal, gastric,* or *esophageal.* Peptic ulcers form at one time or another in about 10 per cent of the population, but only a very small group are diagnosed.

A peptic ulcer will produce pain of a burning or gnawing character felt in the upper abdomen and sometimes also in the back. The pain is generally helped by eating, drinking milk, or taking an alkalinizing medication. Because food helps ulcer pain, the symptoms tend to go away after eating, only to recur several hours later; between-meal pain and discomfort are therefore a common complaint. They can also occur during the night, so that peptic ulcer victims often wake during the night with reactivation of pain. In about 95 per cent of the cases the diagnosis can be proved by taking an X-ray.

Treatment. The treatment of peptic ulcer consists of a bland diet with omission of spices; fried, smoked, or greasy foods; liquor; and preferably also smoking. Neutralization of acids is promoted by small frequent feedings, frequent consumption of milk or milk-cream mixtures, and the taking of alkalinizers which are available in the form of a great many commercial products (Maalox®, Gelusil®, Amphojel®, Titralac®, etc.). One satisfactory program calls for eating some one item in any of these three categories—bland food, milk, alkalizer—every hour throughout the day. If pain recurs regularly at night, an alarm clock may be set so as to wake the sleeper before the expected discomfort, which can then be forestalled by eating, or by drinking milk.

UPPER RESPIRATORY INFECTIONS

▶ **Croup (Acute Laryngotracheobronchitis)** This is an upper respiratory infection due either to virus or bacteria (streptococcus, pneumococcus, staphylococcus). It involves one or more of the structures of the voice box (larynx) and throat. Infants and children have an airway only about the diameter of a pencil. Upper respiratory infections which cause swelling of this area are therefore of a more serious nature than is the case with adults. The infections may involve the tonsils, the lower portion of the trachea, the larynx, and the lungs.

Symptoms. The symptoms of this infection cause difficulty in breathing *in.* This results in a harsh, barking cough and a noisy, groaning inspiration. There may be such difficulty breathing in that the face becomes red and the expression anxious. The skin may turn bluish due to lack of oxygen. The child is "pulling," and the breathing is labored. A great deal of mucus accumulates in the tracheobronchial tree, and the air passages may become obstructed. It is very hard for these infants to cough up mucus. They struggle with both the inability to get air in and the inability to cough up the obstructive phlegm. The stridor (difficult breathing) also manifests itself by retractions at the neck and the sternal notch. Intercostal retractions between the ribs also occur.

Treatment. The two measures which are most useful in relieving the breathing distress are: (1) To place the child in a room or atmosphere filled with warm, moist steam. One method is to turn on the hot shower and hot-water tap in the bathroom, close the door, and sit with the child in this steamy atmosphere for fifteen to twenty minutes. This will usually relieve some of the congestion, and the child will breathe easier. (2) The child can be helped to vomit. This will bring up a great deal of the trapped, thickened mucus. If the child is unable to vomit, he may be given one teaspoon of syrup of ipecac followed by some warm water; your doctor may prescribe a larger dosage for a child over two years old. This is a nauseating agent. If it is given, the child should remain in a seated position so that when he vomits he will not choke on the vomitus.

Children who have been "pulling" or breathing with stridor and difficulty for more than six to eight hours are in danger of exhaustion.

Children with croup should always be seen by a physician. If croup becomes very severe, it may be necessary to operate and perform a tracheotomy. This procedure opens an airway through the trachea (windpipe) below the area of swelling and obstruction. A metal tube is inserted and kept in place, and suctioning of mucus is performed so that the child may breathe with ease. Such cases must usually be hospitalized. When the infection has cleared and the child is able to breathe well by himself, the opening can be closed.

▶ **Strep Throat** This is a throat infection caused by streptococcus. The bacillus can usually be cultured from the throat. Beta-hemolytic streptococcus is the most virulent. It produces toxic substances, high fever, and severe disease. The group A beta-hemolytic streptococcus is responsible for scarlet fever. Streptococci have been implicated in rheumatic fever.

Treatment. Most streptococcus infections can be cured with penicillin and other antibiotics.

VAGINITIS   Vaginitis is any inflammation of the vagina. It generally consists of an annoying discharge, and in severe cases there is pain, burning, itching, and a scalding sensation with the passage of urine. One of the common organisms that may produce this condition is called *Trichomonas,* so that the disorder is sometimes referred to as trichomoniasis.

The organism can sometimes be passed from a woman to her husband and vice versa, so that in stubborn cases both may have to be treated. Various suppositories, insufflation with powders, douches, and a recently developed medication to be taken by mouth may all be used. The infection often flares up after the time of menstruation, and it is generally advisable to continue the treatment through at least two menstrual cycles and even throughout menstruation.

Another form of vaginitis is caused by a fungus known as *Candida,* hence the term candidiasis. This is, perhaps, the most common form of vaginitis to appear during pregnancy. Here too, inflammation may vary from mild to almost intolerable, usually with a thin, somewhat odorous discharge. Another condition which may produce this form of vaginitis is diabetes, since the sugar in the urine favors the growth of the organism. Various suppositories, jellies, and douches may be used in treatment. Both of these organisms may sometimes be found together, producing a mixed form of vaginitis.

Senile vaginitis is sometimes seen in post-menopausal women. At this time, in the absence of hormone treatment, the lining of the vagina is thin and has a low resistance to infection. There may be slight bleeding as well as a discharge which is thin and irritating. One of the most widely employed forms of treatment for this is the use of female hormone, either by suppository or by mouth. This thickens the vaginal lining, increases its resistance, and is generally sufficient to abolish the infection. Occasionally *Trichomonas* and other organisms may be found, and treatment will have to be directed against these organisms. Vaginitis may be most troublesome and annoying, and may call for great patience.

VENEREAL DISEASES   Venereal diseases are generally transmitted by sexual intercourse. The two most common are *gonorrhea* and *syphilis*.

► **Gonorrhea**   The symptoms of gonorrhea appear, on the average, five days after exposure. In the male they consist of a milky-white to yellowish discharge from the penis, with redness and irritation around its opening. In a woman, similar discharge with irritation of the vaginal and urinary channels occurs.

Since various kinds of vaginal discharges and urinary symptoms due to other causes are common in women, a gonorrheal infection may not seem quite so alarming or striking in the female. Also, undoubtedly some of these infections are milder than others. In the more serious forms of the disease an untreated gonorrheal infection may ascend through the uterus and produce considerable inflammation in the tubes and the ovaries. One of the unfortunate consequences of such tubal infection when it heals is that it may produce sterility. In mild cases the doctor may have to do smears or special cultures to determine the existence of gonorrhea.

Gonorrhea responds quite promptly to various sulfa drugs and antibiotics. A vast decrease in the amount of gonorrhea is indicated by the fact that with most men a discharge from the penis will turn out to be "non-specific"—not due to a gonorrheal infection. Very occasionally gonorrhea may be transmitted by a non-venereal route. This is occasionally seen in young children to whom an infection may be transmitted by careless handling by an adult having the disease. The eyes, particularly, are subject to infection with the organism of gonorrhea. In the presence of such an infection scrupulous cleanliness is necessary to avoid a spread.

► **Syphilis**   Syphilis does not produce a discharge but appears first as a local sore. In the male the sore is seen most frequently near the head of the penis, is generally less than dime-sized, and has a moist ulcerated appearance. It is known as a chancre. It will clear up within a few weeks, even without treatment. Since in women the chancre will be internally situated in the vagina or the cervix, it will not be obvious externally. Hence primary syphilis in the female may go completely unnoted. Though the chancre will disappear without treatment, the syphilitic infection will not. Syphilis is notorious for remaining in the system for years without producing evident harm. During this time, however, important organs including the aorta, the large blood vessel leading from the heart, and also the nervous system may become involved. The former may result in syphilitic heart disease, the latter in various forms of paralysis and insanity.

The long silent stage in syphilis that follows the chancre would be most difficult to detect were it not for the important test known as the *Wassermann test* and some of the more recent modifications of this test. Sometimes referred to simply as "a blood test," it is required by law in many states before a marriage certificate can be issued. It is generally routinely done on pregnant women, and indeed is often done as a routine test in hospital admissions. Rather rarely the test may be positive in a person who, one is reasonably sure, never had a syphilitic infection. This is referred to as a biological false-positive. As a rule, however, a positive test generally calls for a course of treatment. Fortunately, since the advent of penicillin and related drugs, the treatment of syphilis has been enormously simplified. Despite successful treatment and eradication of the syphilitic infection, the Wassermann test may remain positive for years thereafter. When this happens, the individual is said to be "Wassermann-fast."

WARTS A wart is a benign (harmless) skin growth and is known to be produced by a virus; why some individuals are susceptible to this virus at certain stages in their lives is not known. Warts are most commonly seen in children and young adults. The most frequent site is on the fingers or the back of the hands, but warts may also occur on the face and, not uncommonly, on the sole of the foot. In the latter location, they tend to be pushed into the skin by one's weight and therefore do not protrude above the surface; these are known as plantar warts. One evidence of the infectious nature of warts is sometimes seen in their distribution in a line which can occur from scratching the original wart and distributing the virus in the line of the scratch.

Treatment. Warts will often disappear spontaneously, the individual waking up one day to find them gone. Another peculiarity of warts is that they are the only form of skin growth known which can disappear by suggestion; painting them with a completely harmless and inert coloring agent may make them disappear if a strong suggestion to this effect is given simultaneously. Occasionally, for large numbers of warts, hypnosis will even be effective. Such suggestion will take one to two weeks, during which time it becomes obvious that the wart is shrinking and being cast off.

Other treatments that have been used include touching the wart with acids, caustic alkalies, or extract of podophyllin; freezing with carbon dioxide ice; and (occasionally) X-ray treatments. A recent suggestion has been the immersion of the wart in hot water (about 116°F.) for half an hour; this hot-water treatment may clear up warts if repeated on a daily basis.

Plantar warts are particularly stubborn because the wart is buried in the skin, often quite deeply. Repeated applications of caustic agents or X-ray treatments may be necessary. Some of the results that are achieved are doubtless due to the self-limited nature of the wart.

WHOOPING COUGH (PERTUSSIS)   Contagious.

Cause. Bacterial, *Hemophilus pertussis.*

Incubation period. 5 days to 3 weeks.

Symptoms. This disease occurs most commonly in January and February in northern climates and in May in southern climates. It may occur at any age but is particularly serious if it occurs in infants below one year of age. In typical cases there is a mild period in the beginning, characterized by a cough which becomes more frequent at night and in the next ten days to two weeks becomes more severe. It develops into a series of repeated spasms of cough, ending in a forced inspiration which is called "the whoop." This is called the spasmodic or paroxysmal stage. Frequently this stage is followed by vomiting or coughing up large amounts of thick mucus. Small infants may turn blue or black from lack of oxygen. In severe cases, they develop nosebleeds or hemorrhages in the eyes due to the great effort of coughing. The disease may last from four to six weeks.

Complications. Bronchitis, bronchopneumonia, etc., are common. Dehydration as a result of prolonged vomiting may occur.

Treatment. Small infants should be hospitalized as they may require oxygen. Antibiotics and hyperimmune serum may be necessary. Sedating cough mixtures help lessen cough spasms.

Prevention. Active immunization of all infants should be started by the third month of age. This consists of an injection of DPT (combined diphtheria, pertussis, tetanus) vaccine. It is usually given in monthly injections for three months, followed by booster doses at one year of age and every three years thereafter. If triple vaccine immunization is not provided, individual immunization with whooping cough vaccine may be given.

The treatment of mild cases is aspirin for the fever and cough medicine to modify the coughing spells. In infants, special care must be taken to prevent their breathing in the vomit and mucus.

WORMS OR PARASITES

Many different types of worms may infest the intestinal tracts. The most common ones are the pinworm, the whipworm, and the roundworm.

Pinworms are white, threadlike worms one-half to three-quarters of an inch long. Their eggs are deposited on the mucous lining and skin around the rectum. The worms may frequently be seen coming out of the rectum and mixed with stool.

Whipworms resemble pinworms but may be larger.

Roundworms are considerably larger, anywhere from six to eight inches long and one-eighth to one-quarter inch in diameter. They are unmistakable.

The symptoms of "worms" vary and may be minimal or severe. There may be no signs or symptoms except vague complaints of poor appetite, poor growth and development, vague abdominal pains, occasional diarrhea, or bloody, tarry stools. Itching or scratching around the rectal area may also be a complaint. If the worms are actually seen, they may be saved and examined. Different worms may require different chemicals for treatment.

A worm which is eaten in uncooked or undercooked pork causes a disease called *trichinosis*. In this condition the eyes become puffy and swollen. There may be a rash, itching, intestinal symptoms, etc. Pork should always be well cooked before serving in order to avoid this condition.

A tropical parasite which does not commonly occur in the United States is the *amoeba* which produces *amoebic dysentery*. This causes severe symptoms of diarrhea, bloody stools, loss of weight, etc. Another worm which occurs in tropical and semi-tropical countries is *hookworm*. It also appears in the southern part of the United States.

The diagnosis of most worm diseases is made by isolating and identifying the worm or its egg in the stool of the patient. It may be necessary to test repeated samples of stool to find eggs or worms. Practically all worm infestations are treatable. However, some are more difficult to cure than others.

WARM-UP EXERCISES

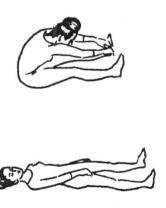

BEND AND STRETCH

Starting position: Stand erect, feet shoulder-width apart.

Action: Count 1. Bend trunk forward and down, flexing knees. Stretch gently in attempt to touch fingers to toes or floor. Count 2. Return to starting position.

Note: Do slowly, stretch and relax at intervals rather than in rhythm.

KNEE LIFT

Starting position: Stand erect, feet together, arms at sides.

Action: Count 1. Raise left knee as high as possible, grasping leg with hands and pulling knee against body while keeping back straight. Count 2. Lower to starting position. Counts 3 and 4. Repeat with right knee.

* Reprinted from United States Adult Physical Fitness Booklet

WARM-UP EXERCISES (Cont'd)

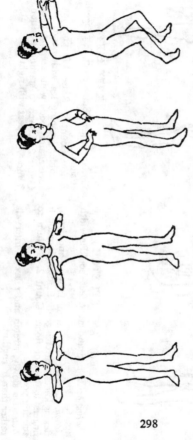

WING STRETCHER

Starting position: Stand erect, elbows at shoulder height, fists clenched in front of chest. *Action:* Count 1. Thrust elbows backward vigorously without arching back. Keep head erect, elbows at shoulder height. Count 2. Return to starting position.

HALF KNEE BEND

Starting position: Stand erect, hands on hips. *Action:* Count 1. Bend knees halfway while extending arms forward, palms down. Count 2. Return to starting position.

WARM-UP EXERCISES (Cont'd)

PRONE ARCH

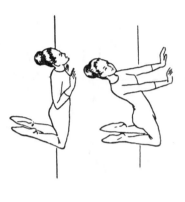

Starting position: Lie face down, hands tucked under thighs.

Action: Count 1. Raise head, shoulders and legs from floor. Count 2. Return to starting position.

KNEE PUSHUP

Starting position: Lie on floor, face down, legs together, knees bent with feet raised off floor, hands on floor under shoulders, palms down.

Action: Count 1. Push upper body off floor until arms are fully extended and body is in straight line from head to knees. Count 2. Return to starting position.

HEAD AND SHOULDER CURL

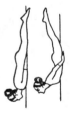

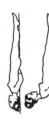

Starting position: Lie on back, hands tucked under small of back, palms down.

Action: Count 1. Tighten abdominal muscles, lift head and pull shoulders and elbows off floor. Hold for four seconds. Count 2. Return to starting position.

WARM-UP EXERCISES (Cont'd)

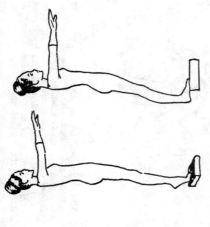

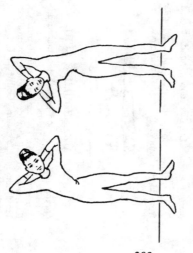

BODY BENDER

Starting position: Stand, feet shoulder-width apart, hands behind neck, fingers interlaced.
Action: Count 1. Bend trunk sideward to left as far as possible, keeping hands behind neck. Count 2. Return to starting position. Counts 3 and 4. Repeat to the right.

ANKLE STRETCH

Starting position: Stand on a stair, large book, or block of wood, with weight on balls of feet and heels raised.
Action: Count 1. Lower heels. Count 2. Raise heels.

FOR THE WAIST

Knee Lifts

Starting position: Lie on back with knees slightly bent, feet on floor and arms at sides.
Action: Count 1—Bring one knee as close as possible to chest, keeping hands on floor. Count 2—Extend leg straight up. Count 3—Bend knee and return to chest. Count 4—Return to starting position. Repeat 5–10 times, alternating legs during exercise.

The double knee lift is done in the same manner, raising both legs at the same time. Do 5–10 repetitions.

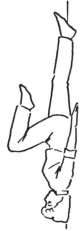

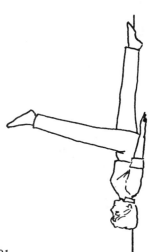

EXERCISES FOR REDUCING AND CONDITIONING

FOR THE BUSTLINE

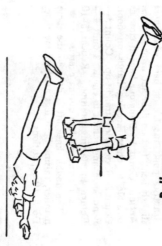

The Press

Starting position: Stand or sit erect. Clasp hands, palms together, close to chest. **Action:** Press hands together hard and hold for 6–8 seconds. Repeat three times, resting briefly and breathing deeply between repetitions.

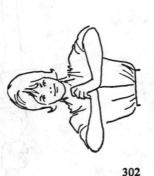

Pullover

Starting position: Lie on back with arms extended beyond head. Hold books or other objects of equal weight in hands. **Action:** Count 1—Lift books overhead and down to thighs, keeping arms straight. Count 2—Return slowly to starting position. Repeat 3–6 times.

Semaphore

Starting position: Lie on back with arms extended sideward at shoulder level. Hold books or other objects of equal weight in hands. **Action:** Count 1—Lift books to position over body, keeping arms straight. Count 2—Lower slowly to starting position. Repeat 3–6 times.

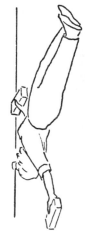

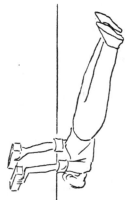

303

INDEX

A

abdomen, distended, 5
abdomen, increased size in
    pregnancy, 5
abdominal pain, 5, 16, 105, 127,
    182, 197, 289
abdominal tumor, 67
abortion, 6, 125
abortive polio, 247
abscess, 7, 57
abscess, amoebic, 8
abscess, appendiceal, 7
abscess, breast, 7
abscess, lung, 7
abscess, pelvic, 8
abscess, teeth, 8
aids, 8
achondroplasia, 239
acidifying salts, 133
acidosis, 107
acne, 263
acne rosacea, 265
ACTH, 209
acute leukemia, 67
acute otitis media, 137
acyanotic heart disease, 198
adenitis, 17
adenoids, 287
ADH, 210
adolescence, 194
adrenal glands, 54, 209
adrenal tissue, 67
after baby arrives, 86-95, 259
afterbirth, 82, 93
afterpains, 92
agammaglobulinemia, 52

aging, effects of, 18, 20, 28, 54,
    132, 256
air passages, obstruction of, 126
air swallowing, 105
albumin, 51
albuminuria, 51
alcohol sponge rub, 9
allergic asthma, 23
allergic diseases of skin, 267
allergy, 10-14, 19, 106, 130, 237,
    267
allergy in children, 10-14, 218
alopecia areata, 28
aluminum salts, 56
alveolar abscess, 8
alveoli, 241
Alzheimer's, 13
ammonia dermatitis, 269
amoebic abscess, 8
amoebic dysentery, 296
anemia, 14-16, 50, 124
anemia in pregnancy, 15
angioma, 41
angioneurotic edema, 269
animal bites and wounds, 43
antibiotics, 129
antibodies, 10, 52
anticoagulants, 104, 130
antidotes, poisoning, 244-46
antigens, 10
antihistamines, 13, 238
antiperspirants, 56
antirabies serum, 249
antirabies vaccine, 249
antirachitic vitamin (vitamin D),
    123
anxiety, 34-35

aphasia, congenital, 194
appendiceal abscess, 7
appendicitis, 6, 7, 16
appendix, 16
appetite, 79
Apresoline, 55
apthous stomatitis, 70
areola, 62
arterial bleeding, 47
arteriosclerosis, 18
artery(ies), hardening of, 18, 54, 95
arthritis, 19
artificial respiration, 22
Aschheim-Zondek test, 74
ascorbic acid (vitamin C), 114, 123
aspirin, 8, 143, 197
asthma, 22
asthmatoid bronchitis, 11, 23, 64
astrocytomas, 58
ataxia, 58
atherosclerosis, 18, 95
athetoid motions, 232
athlete's foot, 265
atropine, 13
A-Z test, 74

B

babies, premature, 84
baby blues, 93
baby care, 84, 96, 105, 118, 123, 144, 177, 185, 204, 212, 215, 216, 234, 263, 269, 274, 278, 285, 289
baby-sitters, 23
backache, 25
backache, abdominal supports for, 26
backbone, fracture of, 142
bacteria, effects on skin, 55, 57
bad bite, 280
bad breath, 56
balance, disorder of, 58
baldness, 27
barbiturates, 132
barbituric acid, 132

base, 107
bath, alcohol sponge rub, 9
bedrest, 91, 104
bed wetting, 34
bee stings, 44
behavior, 28-39
behavior problems in children, 29-38, 59
Bell's palsy, 236
Bender Motor Gestalt test, 221
beriberi, 122
bicarbonate of soda, 198
bile pigments, 15, 201
bile tract, malformations of, 223
biliary colic, 182
bilirubin, 15, 222
biopsy, 63
biotin, 123
birth control, 39-41, 129
birth, multiple, 85
birthmark, 41
bites, 43-44
blackheads (acne), 264
bladder disorders, 45
bladder, urinary, 70
bleeding, 45, 47, 67
bleeding, arterial, 47
bleeding peptic ulcer, 49
bleeding, pressure points, 47
bleeding, severe, 49
blindness, 140
blisters, 65, 73
blood, 50-53
blood, abnormal states of, 14-16, 67
blood cells, 14-16, 50, 222
blood cholesterol, 95
blood clot(ting), 18, 39, 131
blood counts, 50, 67
blood fats, 18
blood platelets, 50
blood pressure, 53-55
blood pressure, drop in, 104
blood pressure, high, 53, 133, 226
blood pressure, low, 53
blood pressure, normal, 53
blood pressure test, 53

blood vessels, 18, 47
body odor, 55
boils, 7, 57
bone age, 193
bone marrow, 51, 65
bones, growth, 192
bones, pelvic, 79
booster shots, 212
bow legs, 239
bowel movements, 102
brachial artery, 47
Braille system, 141
brain, 58
brain concussion, 100
brain disorders, 38, 58-61, 220, 232
brain tumor, 58
brainstem, 58, 247
breast, 62
breast abscess, 7
breast cancer, 68
breast feeding, 86, 216
breath, bad, 56
breathing, difficulty in, 22
breathing rate, 190
breech delivery, 83
bronchi, 63
bronchial tubes, 22, 63
bronchitis, 11, 23, 63
bronchopneumonia, 64, 242
bronchospasm, 22
bruises, 142
bulbar polio, 247
bulk laxatives, 134
burns, 65

C

Caesarian section, 80, 83
calcium, 111, 124
calories, 118
cancer, 65-68, 284
cancer, cervix, 96
cancer, detection, 68
cancer, early warning signals, 68
cancer, penis, 96
Candida, 291

canker sore, 70
capillaries, 41
car sickness, 128
carbuncles, 7, 57
cardiac catheterization, 70
carpopedal spasm, 215
cartilage, 19
castor oil, 134
cat scratch fever, 43
cathartics, 134
catheterization, 70
cauterization, 72
cavernous angioma, 41
celiac syndrome, 71
centers of ossification, 192
cerebellum, 58
cerebral hemispheres, 58
cerebral palsy, 232
cerebrospinal fluid, 58
cervical vertebrae, 273
cervix, 69, 72, 254
chancre, 292
change of life, 228
chemotherapy, 68
chest, 190, 241
chickenpox, 73
child care, 204-08
childbirth afterpains, 92
childbirth and prenatal care, 73-87
childbirth, natural, 82
childhood, 186-96
childhood disorders, 215
children, accident prevention, 8
children, adjustment problems of,
    28-39
children, diet requirements, 119-22
children, mouth-to-mouth
    resuscitation, 22
chlorothiazide, 55, 133
cholecystitis, 182
cholecystokinin, 209
cholelithiasis, 183
cholesterol, 18, 95
chromosomes, 60, 183
chromosomes, sex, 184
chronic bronchitis, 64
chronic cystic mastitis, 62

cigarette smoking, 64, 225, 272
circulation, blood, 18
circulation, impaired, 18, 132
circulatory disorders, 55, 224
circumcision, 96
citrate of magnesia, 134
cleanliness, 55, 261
cleft palate, 215
climacteric, 228
clitoris, 254
clot(ting), blood, 18, 131
club foot, 238
cobalt, 124
coccyx, 272
cold, common, 96
cold compresses, 142
cold-like symptoms, 10-14
colic, 5, 105
colic, biliary, 182
colicky pains, 5, 105
colitis, 98
colon, 98, 127
colostrum, 86
coma, 108
common cold, 96
complete hysterectomy, 211
complex, emotional, 35
compress, 47, 99, 142
compresses, cold, 99
compresses, hot wet, 57, 99
concave lens, 140
concomitant squint, 138
concussion, 100
condom, 40
congenital aphasia, 194
congenital heart disease, 198
conjunctiva, 138
conjunctivitis, 138
constipation, 98, 102
contraception, 39, 72
contracted pelvis, 83
convex lens, 140
convulsion, 103, 233
copper, 124
copperhead bite, 45
coral snake bite, 45
cornea, 139

coronary arteries, 18, 103
coronary thrombosis, 103
cottonmouth bite, 45
cough, 63
coumadin, 131
cradle cap, 269
cramps, 105, 230
cramps, night, 105
creams, contraceptive, 40
crepitus, 141
cretinism, 210
criminal abortion, 7
cross eyes, 138
croup, 289
crowning, 81
cryptorchidism, 256
curettage, 124
curette, 124
cuts, 47
cyanotic heart disease, 198
cystic fibrosis, 71, 106
cystic mastitis, 62
cystitis, 45
cystocele, 46
cystoscopy, 108

D

D and C, 124
dandruff, 266
deciduous teeth, 278
delivery, 80-87, 250
Denis Browne bar, 239
dental abscess, 8
dental hygiene, 56
deodorants, 56
depression, 36, 93
depressive reaction, 36
descending colon, 127
desensitization, 13
development, emotional, 28-29
development, mental, 186-89
development, physical, 186-94
diabetes, 140
diabetes mellitus, 107
diabetic coma, 108

diaper rash, 110, 269
diapers, care of, 109
diaphragm (contraceptive), 40, 72
diarrhea, 71, 98, 110
diastolic blood pressure, 53
dicumarol, 131
diet, 77, 95, 111-24
diet, basic food guide, 113
diet, bland, 98
diet, children's, 119-22
diet, crash, 112
diet deficiency, 111-24
diet, formula, 113
diet, high protein, 116
diet, low calorie, 116
diet, nursing mothers, 88
diet, prudent, 115
diet, reducing, 115-19
diet, special, 71
dietary deficiencies, 122-24
differential growth, 192
diffuse goiter, 283
digestive disturbances, 71
digestive tract, 127, 132
digestive tract hormone, 209
dilatation and curettage, 125
dilation, 124
diphtheria, 125
discharges, vaginal, 39, 92
discipline, 29-32
dislocation, 239
diuretics, 55, 133
diverticula, 126
diverticulitis, 126
dizziness, 128
DNA, 183
dog bites, 43
douches, 129
Down's syndrome, 60
dreams, 34
dropsy, 224
drug allergy, 10-14, 130
drugs and remedies, 129-36
dry bronchitis, 64
dry pleurisy, 241
dry skin, 262
duodenal ulcer, 289

dysentery, 110
dysmenorrhea, 230

E

ear, external, 137
ear infection, 137
ear, inner, 128, 137
ear, middle, 137
eardrum, 137
eclampsia, 51
eczema, 267
edema, 51, 78, 224
electric shock, 261
electrocardiograph, 108
electroencephalogram, 109, 233
embryo, 6, 76, 215
emotional disturbances, 28-39
emotional health, 28-39
emotional stimulus, 28
emotions, 28-39
emotions and allergy, 14
empyema, 241
encephalitic polio, 247
encephalitis, 60, 227
endocervitis, 72
endocrine diseases, 210
endocrine glands, 209
enemas, 206
engorgement, 86
enuresis, 34
enzymes, pancreatic, 106
eosinophils, 51
ephedrine, 132
epididymis, 256
epilepsy, 233
episiotomy, 80, 81
Epsom Salts, 134
equilibrium, 52
ergotamine, 197
erosions, 72
erythroblastosis fetalis, 223
esophageal ulcer, 289
esophagus, 203
essential hypertension, 54
estrogen, 209

excretion, 55
exercise, 26, 94
exocrine glands, 106
exophthalmic goiter, 284
exophthalmos, 211
external hemorrhoids, 200
extroversion, 36
eye, 138-41
eyeglasses, 140

F

fainting, 141
Fallopian tubes, 215
falls, 141
false labor, 80
farsightedness, 140
fats, 19, 71, 95
fats, blood, 18
fear, 33, 34, 82
febrile disease, 234
feeble-mindedness, 222
feeding, breast, 86, 216
feeding of baby, 144, 177-82
female hormones, 104, 143, 209, 229
female sex organs, 254
femoral artery, 49
femoral hernia, 203
fertility, 40
fertilization, 40
fetal development, 76, 215
fetus, 6
fever, 9, 142
fever, high, 9
fibroid tumor, 143, 211
first aid, 144-176
first degree burn, 65
flat feet, 239
flu, 218
fluid retention, 54, 133, 224
fluorides, 279
focal signs, 59
folic acid, 123
folic acid deficiency, 15
fontanelle, 193

food allergy, 10-14, 106
food, basic requirements, 113, 120, 122-24
food deficiencies, 122-24
foot problems, 238
foreskin, 96
formula, preparing, 144, 177-82
fracture, 141
fraternal twins, 85
freckles, 42
Friedman-Lapham test, 74
frigidity, 258
"frog" test, 74
functional colitis, 98

G

gallbladder, 182
gallbladder, infected, 182
gallstones, 182
gamma globulin, 51, 202
gastric ulcer, 289
gastro-intestinal allergy, 12
gavage feeding, 85
genes, 183
genital hygiene, 185
genito-urinary diseases, 185
German measles, 227
gland, swelling of, 231
glands, 209
glands, abdominal, 17
glands, breast, 62
glands, lymph, 43
glandular defects, 106
glandular disorders, 27
gliadin, 71
glioma, 58
globulins, 51
glucose tolerance test, 107
gluten, 71
glycerin suppositories, 278
glycogen, 107
gnat bite, 43
goiter, 283
gonadotropic hormones, 209
gonadotropins, 73

gonorrhea, 292
gouty arthritis, 19
grand mal, 233
Graves' disease, 211
griping pain, 5
griseofulvin, 130
growth and development, 186-96
growth and development, critical
    norms, 186-89

H

hair loss, 27
halitosis, 56
hardening of the arteries, 18, 95
harelip, 215
hay fever, 12, 23, 237
head, distention of, 58
head, growth of, 193
head injuries, 100
headache, 196
hearing, difficulty in, 136
heart, 54, 103
heart attack, 55
heart disease, congenital, 198
heart muscle, 54
heart, palpitation of, 240
heartburn, 197
heartrate, 190
heat exhaustion, 199
heat stroke, 199
heating pad, 99
height, 189
hematoma, 100
hemiplegia, 232
hemoglobin, 14-16, 50
hemoglobin determination test,
    15, 50
hemolytic anemia, 15
hemolytic diseases, 223
hemophilia, 49
hemorrhage, 49
hemorrhoids, 200, 277
heparin, 131
hepatitis, 201
heredity, 27, 49, 60, 183

hernia, 84, 202
herniorrhaphy, 203
herpes simplex, 70
hexachlorophene, 55
hiatus hernia, 203
high blood pressure, 53-54, 133,
    226
hip, dislocation, 239
histamine, 13
hives, 269
Hodgkin's disease, 66
home care, 204-08
hookworm, 296
hormone reaction, 238
hormone treatments, 229
hormones, 19, 27, 73, 86, 135, 143,
    209
hospital, preparing child for, 208
hot flushes, 228
hot-water bottle, 99
humidity, home, 64
hydrocephalus, 59
hydrocortisone, 209
hydrophobia, 248
hygiene, 56
hymen, 254
hyperactivity, 59
hypercholesterolemia, 95
hyperhydrosis, 55
hypermetropia, 140
hypersensitivity, 10-14, 23, 44
hypertension, 53-55, 133
hyperthyroidism, 211, 284
hypervitaminosis, 122
hypoparathyroidism, 210
hypothyroidism, 210, 285
hysterectomy, 144, 211

I

ice bag, 99
icterus neonatorum, 222
icterus praecox, 223
identical twins, 85
idiots, I.Q. of, 222

illness, care of, 9, 97, 99, 106, 199, 200, 204-08, 234, 274, 290
imbeciles, I.Q. of, 222
immunity, 52
immunization, 126, 212
immunization, passive, 126
immunization, record, 214
impaction, 250
impetigo contagiosa, 267
impotence, 255
incarcerated hernia, 203
incision, 45
induced abortion, 7
infancy, 186-94, 263
infancy, emotions in, 28
infancy, recognizing illness in, 207
infant care, 109, 204-08
infant disorders, 100, 215, 234, 269
infant feeding, 144, 177-82, 216-18
infantile tetany, 215
infection, 57, 130
infection, prevention of, 52
infectious hepatitis, 201
infectious mononucleosis, 51, 231
infertility, 276
inflammation, skin, 57
influenza, 218
inguinal canal, 202
inguinal hernia, 202
INH, 130
inheritance of disease, 101
innominate bone, 79
inoculation, 212
insect bites, 43
insecurity, 28-39
insomnia, 132, 219
insulin, 107, 209
insulin shock, 108
intelligence quotient (I.Q.), 222
intelligence tests, 220
intercostal spaces, 241
internal bleeding, 49
internal hemorrhoids, 200
interrupted pregnancy, 6
intertrigo, 269
intestinal obstruction, 5, 215

intestinal pain, 5
intestinal sulfonamides, 136
intestines, 17, 98, 127
intradermal test, 14
introversion, 36
intussusception, 215
involution, 90
iodine, 124
iodine-deficiency goiter, 284
iris, 139
iron, 124
iron deficiency, 14-16
iron deficiency anemia, 16
iron in hemoglobin, 14
iron replenishment, 15
iron supplements, 15
irritant cathartics, 134
itching, 43-44, 263-69

J

jaundice, 15, 201, 222
joint diseases, 19
joints, pain in, 19
joints, thickening of, 20
junctional nevus, 42

K

ketone bodies, 108
kidney, 51, 68
kidney disorders, 51, 54, 185, 225
knock knee, 239
Koplik's spots, 227
kwashiorkor, 120

L

labia majora, 254
labia minora, 254
labor, 80-82
labyrinthitis, 128
laceration, 47
large intestine, 98, 127

laryngitis, 223
larynx, 223
laxatives, 17, 134
left ventricle, 54
leg, 105, 224
lens, corrective, 140
lesions, 41, 70
leukemia, 50, 67
liver, 51
liver inflammations, 201
lobar pneumonia, 242
lobes, 63
lochia, 90, 92
lockjaw, 282
longevity, 225
low back pain, 25
lumbar vertebrae, 273
lung, abscess, 7
lymph glands, swelling of, 43
lymph nodes, 66
lymphatic system, 66
lymphocytes, 50, 67
lymphogranulomatosis, 66
lymphoid tissue, 286

M

magnesium, 124
male hormones, 209
male sex organs, 255
malignant goiter, 284
malignant tumor, 66
malnutrition, 16, 71, 120, 122-24
malocclusion, 280
mammotropic hormone, 209
manganese, 124
mask of pregnancy, 43
mastitis, 62
mastoid, 137
mastoiditis, 137
masturbation, 226
measles, 226
measles, German, 227
Meckel's diverticulum, 127
medication, giving child, 205
medulloblastomas, 58

megacolon, congenital, 100
megaloblastic erythropeosis, 123
melanoma, 42
Meniere's syndrome, 128
meninges, 61
meningitis, 61
menopause, 143, 211, 228
menstrual cycle, 39, 229
menstrual irregularities, 230
menstrual odors, 56
menstruation, 229
menstruation, cessation of, 228
mental and emotional health,
    28-39
mental attitude, 28-39
mental depression, 36
mental diseases and disorders,
    33-38
mental retardation, 60, 210, 220
meprobamate, 136
mercurial diuretics, 133
mesenteric adenitis, 17
metabolic disorders, 19, 101, 106,
    107
metastasis, 66
metatarsus varus, 240
migraine, 197
miliaria, 270
milk of magnesia, 198
milk teeth, 278
minerals in diet, 119-20, 122-24
miscarriage, 6
Mittelschmerz, 230
moles, 42
mongolism, 60
monilia, 215
monocytes, 67
mononucleosis, infectious, 51, 231
monoplegia, 232
morning sickness, 77-78
morons, I.Q. of, 222
mosquito bite, 43
motion sickness, 128
mouth, disturbances, 70
mouth hygiene, 56
mouth-to-mouth resuscitation, 22
mucous membranes, 67

mucus, 64, 97, 289
multiple birth, 85
multiple sclerosis, 237
mumps, 231
mumps serum, 232
muscle cramps, 105
muscle cramps, night, 105
muscular control, diseases
  affecting, 232
muscular dystrophy, 233
myelocytes, 67
myomectomy, 144
myopia, 140

N

nail biting, 34
nasal congestion, 237
nasal passages, 97
natural childbirth, 82
nausea, 77, 233
navel, 84
neck, stiff, 235
nephritis, 185
nephrosis, 185, 225
nephrotic syndrome, 51
nerve cells, 67
nerve, inflammation of, 236
nervous symptoms, 34
nervous system, disorders of, 232,
  248
neuritis, 236
neuroblastoma, 67
neurodermatitis, 267
neurological and neuromuscular
  disorders, 236
neurosis, 33
niacin, 123
nicotinic acid, 123
night cramps, 105
night terrors, 34
nipple, 62, 86-87
nocturnal emission, 196
nodular goiter, 284
non-productive cough, 64
non-toxic goiter, 283

nose, 237
nose drops, 97, 238
nosebleed, 47
nostrils, 97
nucleus pulposus, 273
nursing, 87-90
nursing mother's diet, 88-89
nutrition, 111-24
nutritional anemias, 16
nutritional deficiencies, 71, 122-24
nystagmus, 58

O

oatmeal bath, 277
odors, 55
oil glands, 263
oligomenorrhea, 230
oral contraceptive (the pill), 39
orgasm, 257
orthopedic conditions, 238
orthostatic albuminuria, 51
os, 72, 255
ossification, 192
osteoarthritis, 20
osteoporosis, 112, 274
otitis, 137
ovarian hormones, 143
ovaries, 255
ovaries, removal of, 211
overweight, 226
ovulation, 40, 230, 274
ovum, 255
oxygen, 103
oxytocin, 210

P

pain, abdominal, 5, 16, 105, 127,
  182, 197, 289
pain, back, 25
pain, breast, 63
pain, burns, 65
pain, chest, 241
pain, coronary thrombosis, 104

pain, ear, 137
pain, headache, 197
pain, joint, 19
pain, labor, 80
pain, menstrual, 230
pain, neck, 235
pain, relief of, 25, 65, 86, 99, 106, 200, 241, 277
palpitation, heart, 240
pancreatic enzymes, 106
pancreatic hormone, 209
pantothenic acid, 124
Pap smear test, 69, 72
paralytic squint, 138
paraplegia, 232
parasites, 295
parathyroid gland, 210
paroxysmal fibrillation, 240
paroxysmal tachycardia, 240
passive immunization, 126
passive transfer, 14
Pasteur treatment, 43
patch test, 14
pellagra, 123
pelvic abscess, 8
pelvic outlet, 80
pelvis, 79, 83
penicillin, 129
penicillin allergy, 130
penis, 96, 255
peptic ulcer, 288
peptic ulcer, bleeding, 49
perianal dermatitis, 270
periodontitis, 279
peritonitis, 17
permanent teeth, 278
personality, 37, 59
perspiration, 56
pertussis, 294
pessary, 46
petit mal, 233
phenobarbital, 132
phenylalanine, 101
phenylketonuria, 101
pheochromocytomas, 54
Philadelphia chromosome, 60
phimosis, 96

phlegm, 63-64
phobia, 33
phosphorus, 124
phospho-soda, 134
physical allergy, 238
physiologic jaundice, 222
pigmentation, 42
pimples (acne), 264
pinkeye, 138
pinworm, 295
pituitary gland, 209
pituitary hormones, 86, 209
PKU, 101
plantar warts, 293
plasma cells, 50
platelets, 50
play therapy, 39
pleura, 241
pleural effusion, 241
pleurisy, 241
pleuritis, 241
pneumonia, 64, 241
pneumonia, lobar, 242
pneumonia, virus, 242
poison ivy, 242
poison oak, 242
poison sumac, 242
poisonous snakes, 45
poisons, 5, 244-46
poliomyelitis, 247
pollen, hay fever, 10-14
polydypsia, 107
polymenorrhea, 230
polymorphonuclear leukocytes, 50
polyneuritis, 236
polyphagia, 107
polyunsaturated fats, 19, 104
polyuria, 107
port-wine mark, 42
postconcussive syndrome, 100
posterior fontanelle, 193
posterior fossa, 58
post-partum care, 86-94
posture, 94
potassium, 124, 133
pregnancy, 5, 43, 62, 73-87, 105, 219, 224, 228, 260

pregnancy, anemia in, 15
pregnancy, eclampsia in, 51
pregnancy, interrupted, 6
pregnancy tests, 73
premature babies, 84
prenatal care, 77
presbyopia, 140
pressure, high blood, 53-55, 133
pressure, low blood, 53
pressure points, 47
prickly heat, 270
primary syphilis, 292
primary tuberculosis, 287
primordial follicles, 255
progesterone, 209
prostate gland, 255
protein deficiency, 120
proteins, 119
protoscopy, 108
psoriasis, 267
psychoanalysis, 39
psychological speech defects, 195
psychological tests, 59
psychopathic personality, 37
psychosis, 38
psychosomatic disorders, 14, 132
psychotherapy, 37, 38
puberty, 195, 263
pubic bones, 79
pubic symphysis, 79
pulmonic circulation, 198
pulse, 248
punishment, 32-34
pupil, 139
purgative, 134
pus, 57
pyelitis, 185
pyloric stenosis, 101
pyorrhea, 279
pyridoxine (vitamin B₆), 124

Q

quadriplegia, 232

R

"rabbit" test, 74
rabies, 248
ragweed, 13
rashes, 10-14, 73, 227, 252, 263-71
rattlesnake bite, 45
rauwolfia, 55
reading glasses, 140
recognizing illness in infants, 207
rectocele, 47
rectum, 47, 250
red blood cell determination test,
    15
red blood cells, 50
red blood cells, diseases of,
    14-16, 222
reducible hernia, 202
reducing diet, 115-19
respiration, 248
respiration, artificial, 22
respiratory diseases, 64, 289
respiratory rate, 248
retardation, mental, 60
retention of fluid, 54, 133, 224
retina, 140
RH disease, 223
rheumatic fever, 251
rheumatoid arthritis, 20
rhinitis, 238
rhythm method, 40
riboflavin (vitamin B₂), 122
rickets, 123, 239
ringworm, 268
Rorschach test, 221
roseola infantum, 270
roundworm, 295
rubella, 227
rubeola, 226

S

sacral vertebrae, 273
sacroiliac, 25
safe period, 40
saline cathartics, 134

salivary glands, 231
saturated fats, 19
scabies, 268
scarlatina, 251
scarlet fever, 251
Schick test, 126
schizophrenia, 38
sciatica, 236
scoliosis, 273
scorpion bite, 44
scratch test, 13
scrotum, 255
scurvy, 123
sea-sickness, 128
seasonal asthma, 23
sebaceous glands, 266
seborrheic dermatitis, 124, 266, 269
second degree burn, 65
secondary anemia, 71
secretin, 209
secretions, 54
secretions, eye, 138
sedatives, barbiturate, 132
Seidlitz powders, 134
semicircular canals, 128
seminal vesicle, 255
sensitivity (allergy), 10-14
sepsis with jaundice, 223
septum, 47
serum hepatitis, 201
serum sickness, 12
sex education, 252
sex glands, 231
sex hormones, 19, 209, 262
sex organs, 254-56
sexual harmony, 256
sexual intercourse, 92, 259
shingles, 236
shock, electric, 261
shunt, 60
sick care, 9, 97, 99, 106, 199-200, 204-08, 234, 274, 290
sick child, 204-08, 290
sick room, 206
sight, 138, 191
silver nitrate, 139

sitz bath, hot, 200
skin care, 261
skin discoloration, 41
skin disorders, 57
skin disturbances, 263-71
skin eruptions, 242
skin, infant, 263
skin, premature aging, 262
skin tests, allergy, 13
sleeplessness, 219
sleep-producing drugs, 132
sleep requirements, 191
small intestine, 127
smallpox, 271
smegma, 96
smell, sense of, 191
smoking, 64, 226, 271
snakebite, 44
soap, 261
sodium, 124
"soft" spots, 193
solid foods, introducing, 217
somatotropic hormone, 209
spasm, 5, 45, 103
spasmophilia, 215
spastic colitis, 98
spastic colon, 98
spasticity, 232
speech, 190, 194
speech defects, psychological, 195
sperm, 40, 256
spermatic cords, 256
spermatogenesis, 256
sphincter, 250
spider bites, 44
spider, black widow, 44
spider, brown recluse, 44
spider nevi, 41
spinal column, 272
spinal disorders, 273
spinal paralytic polio, 247
spinal tap, 61
spine, 25
spine, curvature of, 273
spine, fracture of, 142
spleen, 16, 51, 66
splints, 142

sponge rub, alcohol, 9
spontaneous abortion, 6
sprains, 142
squint, 138
staining, vaginal, 39
standard clean sterilization,
  formula, 180
staphylococcus, 57
starch bath, 277
starches, 71
steam inhalation, 274
sterility, 231, 275
sterilization, formula, 179-82
steroid drugs, 13
steroid hormones, 135
stiff neck, 235
stool-softeners, 134
strabismus, 138
strawberry angioma, 42
strep throat, 290
streptomycin, 129
striae, 6
stroke, 18, 55
sty, 139
subdural hematoma, 100
sulfa drugs, 130, 135
sulfonamides, 130, 135
sulfur, 124
sun, exposure to, 262, 277
sunburn, 276
suppositories, 135, 277
supracervical hysterectomy, 211
surgical menopause, 211
sweat, 55
sweat electrolyte test, 106
synovium, 19
syphilitic jaundice, 223
syphilis, 293
systemic circulation, 198
systolic blood pressure, 53

T

talipes equinovarus, 238
tannic acid, 65
tantrum, 30, 32

target organ, 98, 209
taste, 191
teeth, 278-81
teeth, abscess, 8
teeth, care of, 279
teeth, child's, 278
teething, 279
temper tantrums, 30, 32
temperament, 29
temperature, 281
temperature reduction, 9, 142, 199
temporary immunity, 212
temporary teeth, 278
tendonitis, 19
tension headache, 197
tentorium, 58
terminal sterilization, formula,
  179
terramycin, 130
testes, 255
testicles, 255
testicles, undescended, 256
testosterone, 209, 256
tests, allergy, 13
tests, blood, 14-16, 17
tetanus, 282
tetany, 210
tetracycline, 129
thematic apperception test, 222
therapeutic abortion, 7
thermometer, 281
thiamine chloride (vitamin B_1),
  122
third degree burn, 65
thoracic vertebrae, 273
thorazine, 136
throat spasm, 103
thrombin, 49
thrombocytopenic purpura, 50
thromboplastinogen, 49
thrombosed hemorrhoid, 200
thrombosis, 18, 103, 131
thrush, 215
thumb sucking, 282
thyroid cancer, 284
thyroid deficiency, 210
thyroid gland, 209

317

thyroid gland disorders, 210, 283
thyroiditis, 285
thyroxin, 209
tinea circinata, 268
tissues, swelling of, 51
toilet training, 28, 34, 285
tonsillectomy, 286
tonsillitis, 286
tonsils, 286
torticollis, 235
touch, sensation of, 191
tourniquet, 45, 49
toxemia, 78
toxic adenoma, 211
toxic goiter, 211, 283
trachea, 63
tracheobronchitis, 63
tracheotomy, 126, 290
tranquilizing drugs, 136
trauma, 29
trial of labor, 80
trichinosis, 295
trichomonas, 291
triglycerides, 18
truss, 203
TSH, 209
tubal insufflation test, 276
tuberculin test, 288
tuberculosis, 287
tumor, 58, 66-68, 143
tumor, fibroid, 143
twins, 86

U

ulcer, peptic, 49, 288
umbilical cord, 84
umbilical hernia, 84, 202
undescended testicles, 256
unsaturated fats, 115
upper respiratory infection,
    allergy, 11
upper respiratory infections, 289
uric acid, 19
urinalysis, 51

urinary bladder, 70
urinary tract infections, 185
urination, difficulties in, 34, 45,
    70, 185
urticaria, 267, 269
uterine contractions, 80
uterus, 5, 80, 90, 124, 143, 211,
    229, 254

V

vaccination, 271
vagina, 46, 254
vaginal discharges, 39, 92, 129
vaginal douche, 129
vaginal jellies, creams and
    foams, 40
vaginal suppositories, 278
vaginitis, 129, 291
valvular lesions, 199
varicella, 73
variola, 271
vascular headache, 197
vascular system, 54
veins, distended, 200
venereal disease, 292
ventricle, left, 54
vernix casiosa, 263
vertebrae, 272
vertigo, 128
viral hepatitis, 201
virus pneumonia, 242
vision, disturbance of, 58
vitamin A, 114, 122
vitamin B_1, 122
vitamin B_2, 122
vitamin B_6, 124
vitamin B_{12}, 124
vitamin C, 114, 123
vitamin D, 123
vitamin deficiency, 15, 122-23
vitamin K, 123, 131
vomiting, 77, 101, 233
vulva, 254

W

walking pneumonia, 242
warts, 293
Wasserman test, 293
Wechsler intelligence scale, 220
weight, 190
weight gain, 79
wet dreams, 196
wet pleurisy, 241
wheat sensitivity, 71
wheezing, 22, 64
whipworm, 295
white blood cell determination
   test, 50
white blood cells, 50

white blood cells, diseases of, 67
whooping cough, 294
Wilm's tumor, 68
windpipe, 63
winter itch, 262
womb, 254
worms, intestinal, 295
wry neck, 235

X Y Z

X chromosomes, 184
XX genetic makeup, 184
XY genetic makeup, 184
Y chromosomes, 184
zinc, 124